Family Homeopathy

Keats titles of related interest

The Bach Flower Remedies
    Edward Bach, M.D. and F. J. Wheeler, M.D.

Handbook of the Bach Flower Remedies
    Dr. Philip M. Chancellor

Complementary Natural Prescriptions for Common Ailments
    Carolyn Dean, M.D.

Homeopathic Medicine Today
    Trevor M. Cook, Ph.D.

Homeopathy in Practice
    Douglas Borland, M.D.

The Medical Discoveries of Edward Bach, Physician
    Nora Weeks

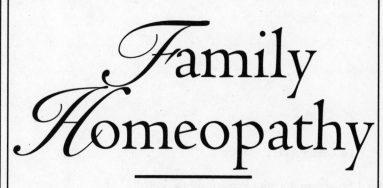

Family Homeopathy

A practical handbook for home treatment

PAUL CALLINAN

Foreword by CAROLYN DEAN, M.D.

Keats Publishing, Inc. New Canaan, Connecticut

FAMILY HOMEOPATHY

Published by arrangement with Penguin Books Australia Ltd
Copyright © 1995 by Paul Callinan
All Rights Reserved

Library of Congress Cataloging-in-Publication Data

Callinan, Paul.
    Family homeopathy: a practical handbook for home treatment / Paul
Callinan, foreword by Carolyn Dean.
        p. cm.
    Includes bibliographical references and index.
    ISBN 0-87983-687-3
    1. Homeopathy—Popular works. 2. Homeopathy—Matoria medica and
therapeutics. I. Title.
RX76.C35 1995
615.5'32—dc20   95-25132
                                                                      CIP

Printed in the United States of America

Published by Keats Publishing, Inc.
27 Pine Street, Box 876
New Canaan, Connecticut 06840-0876

95 96 97 98 6 5 4 3 2 I

Dedication

To my children, Ariel, Damon and Imagene, for
enduring the ministrations of a homeopath.

Disclaimer

The material here is condensed from journals, text-books, research material and clinical experience. The greatest possible care has been taken to insure that it is accurate and complete. However, the medicines and dosages described in this book are offered as guidelines, subject to current knowledge, research findings, the symptoms presented in the case and the individual user's judgment. The author and publishers cannot be held responsible for the misuse of the information, nor for any effects arising from the inappropriate prescription of any of the medicines mentioned. In any treatment program regular contact with a practitioner is recommended.

Acknowledgments

Sincere thanks to Brauer Biotherapies and Martin and Pleasance for their support and encouragement in the writing of this book.

Contents

PART THREE

A Materia Medica of Common Remedies

Foreword

Paul Callinan is an Australian who has a great affinity for homeopathy. He is also a naturopath and chiropractor. But I suspect his first love is homeopathy.

When I sent out a request on the Internet for feedback on this man, I got some glowing praise and the hint of a true explorer, a man pushing the envelope. But part of the glue keeping the envelope together is his attention to the scientific method. The first chapter *Explaining Homeopathy* is a thorough reporting of the studies that prove homeopathy works and that its benefits are not due to placebo effect. For those of us who already know that homeopathy works because we have had first hand experience, this may not be necessary; however, in order for the practice of homeopathy to spread and be accepted by the medical profession, these studies are essential.

I was also very impressed with Dr. Callinan's ability to synthesize the recent advances in biophysics, hormesis and pharmacology in a successful attempt to explain how and why homeopathy works. Back in 1888 Arndt developed the Arndt-Schulz Law, which stated that for every substance, small doses stimulate, moderate doses inhibit, large doses kill. The world followed the path of moderate drug doses, which work on the inhibitory curve of the scale producing the suppressant effect of drugs. Homeopathic medicine begins at the lower doses which are stimulatory and moves to even smaller doses. This is in an effort to stimulate the body's natural balancing mechanisms.

Hormesis is the Arndt-Schulz Law revived in modern toxicology. Since 1960 data has demonstrated the existence of two effects of poisonous substances on living organisms. At high doses they inhibited metabolism and ultimately caused death, but at low doses they exerted a stimulating effect. This is an astonishing finding and parallels the action of homeopathy. At large doses a drug can cause the same symptoms that can be treated with small doses.

Dr. Callinan also explains the mechanism by which the water molecules are imprinted with the vibratory rate of the substance being potentized. He explains that this work is in the realm of biophysics, that it is a relatively new discipline and that most medical doctors are not familiar with it and therefore ignore or deny its findings. Biophysics can apply tests to water which determine that structural changes do occur in water when a substance is diluted and succussed. When water alone, with no substance added, is succussed, there are no structural changes. It is this change in the water molecule that imparts information to the body to cause a desired effect.

Thus far I have only talked about one chapter of a very large homeopathic encyclopedia. The rest of the book is just as impressive. Callinan has managed to include, not only a homeopathic *materia medica*, but also a complete review of the Bach Flower Remedies, the 12 tissue salts, a first-aid kit and comprehensive treatments for 130 conditions.

The Bach Flower Remedies were one of the first modalities that I learned, and I found them invaluable in practice. Dr. Callinan has managed to transmit the essence of each remedy in a very brief description that can be easily memorized and be recalled to treat specific conditions as they arise.

The 12 tissue salts are low-potency homeopathics of mineral salts that seem to work because they treat a mineral deficiency in the patient but they also have a particular homeopathic picture that Dr. Callinan describes very clearly.

The *materia medica* listing of remedies is also described in a most concise and "user-friendly" way. The keynotes of the remedy and general appearance of the patient who needs the remedy are set apart from the symptom picture, which makes it much easier to understand what to prescribe. In most old texts all three aspects are often jumbled together and it is hard to get the feel of a remedy. It is wise to read through this section to familiarize yourself with the remedies that seem to suit you, your disposition and tendencies, so that when the need arises you are able to go straight to a short list of possibilities. It is this type of knowledge that centers you and allows you to focus on helping yourself or your family. There is no better resource or means of taking responsibility for your health than homeopathy.

The therapy section itself comprises the bulk of the book. There are chapters on first aid, common ailments, infants, children, mothers, women and men. For each condition there are from two to 20 remedies prescribed and often a little naturopathic advice thrown in for good measure.

The chapter for mothers is comprehensive and includes such difficult problems as herpes in pregnancy and miscarriage. The miscarriage section covers threatened and true miscarriage and delineates the different remedies for both. There is a detailed section on labor which should be extremely helpful to any doctor, midwife or mother. There are no natural allopathic treatments for easing labor. What a wonderful way to bring a new life into the world with the use of natural, nontoxic homeopathic remedies.

Dr. Callinan has done a great service in writing this exceptional book. *Family Homeopathy* will replace several books that I previously used for reference.

Family Homeopathy is a wonderful book for the novice lay homeopath and a great reference book for the knowledgeable. I recommend it highly.

Carolyn Dean, B.Sc., M.D.

Introduction

HOMEOPATHY: ITS PLACE IN MEDICINE

Homeopaths, like all natural therapists, have always agreed on the most fundamental point in the treatment of disease: that disease is caused by mistakes in the habits of living. Correct the mistakes of living, the thinking goes, and disease will take care of itself. Only if the body has trouble in regaining its equilibrium should medicine be given.

To date, this approach to medicine has served us well. It has taken the responsiblity for personal health from the doctor and given it back to the individual. The message has been clear: live well, and last longer; look after your life, and its quality will improve. Our vitality, a precious gift, should be nurtured; our life should be in our own hands.

Vitality is the health factor that orthodox medicine has forgotten. Known more correctly as **allopathy**, orthodox medicine is just one of the ten or so mainstream schools of medical thought existing throughout the world: massage, herbalism, nature cure, nutrition, naturopathy, ayurveda, unani, acupuncture, osteopathy, chiropractic and homeopathy make up the list of the main alternative medicines. These systems are traditionally developed, with their roots deep in their countries' cultures. A number, like acupuncture and ayurveda, go back several thousand years.

Homeopathy is a newcomer, as it goes back only two hundred years, to a time when allopathy was already flourishing in Europe. It was developed in Germany, although both homeopathy and allopathy claim their roots in Hippocrates, a Greek of the late fifth century BC, generally acknowledged to be the father of modern medicine. Hippocrates, in turn, had already been influenced by unani, the medicine of the ancient Persians and Egyptians, and by ayurveda from India. In this way it can be seen that many medical systems have common beginnings.

Most of these medicines, with the notable exception of allopathy, have as their basic tenet that it is the vital energy of the patient that must be treated, not just the physical symptoms. These medical systems are currently used for the treatment of well over half of the world's population, and many have the support of the World Health Organization, particularly in Third World countries. This support is fostering research, and an emergence of traditional medicines is occurring worldwide.

The great developments that allopathic medicine lists as proof of its effectiveness are mostly confined to the development of sophisticated tests, the treatment of life-threatening disorders, such as infection and traumatic injury, and to one of its greatest triumphs, essential surgery. In these areas it is without peer. Much of this development began in World War II, when the need for these was high; the development of specialized surgical procedures, antibiotics and pain killers were particularly notable achievements. It was believed these successes would be repeated with breakthroughs in the treatment of a broader range of illnesses.

But the routine use of allopathic medicines in treatment is not showing the success hoped for; the cost of drug research is going up, and reports of side effects are increasing. The public is becoming more aware of the toxic effects of many drugs. It is no news to anyone acquainted with the allopathic system that it functions principally to treat existing illness and to care for the chronically ill: to pull people out of the river and resuscitate them, rather than to prevent them falling in. There is a neglect of *prevention*, and the incidence of most preventable diseases (such as cancer, asthma, heart disease, osteoporosis and hypertension) remains unacceptably high. There is also a lack of urgency in the treatment of chronic disease compared with acute disease; with the exception of injuries, Western medicine's most prevalent, serious, and costly health problems nearly all concern chronic disease.

Homeopathy is regarded by its practitioners as being well suited to the treatment of most common disorders, including chronic disease, where allopathy is less appropriate. Homeopathic medicines offer many advantages, the greatest being that they are safe, easy to use and cheap. Homeopathy is a system of medicine easily understood by the lay person, and one of its greatest uses is in the treatment of domestic ailments.

HOMEOPATHIC MEDICINES

The medicines are usually sold either as liquids or in pillules of calcium lactate, otherwise known as sugar of milk. An alcohol-and-water mixture is the most common liquid form, and most prescriptions in this book will be for liquid, although a few different preparations exist.

Mother tinctures are concentrated extracts, in an alcohol and water base. They can be made from any substance in the animal, vegetable or mineral kingdoms. All told, probably about 2000 homeopathic mother tinctures have been prepared from different substances, and more are always being tested somewhere in the world. Mother tinctures are used as raw material, and in homeopathy are seldom used undiluted, except occasionally on wounds. The proportion of alcohol, which is used as a preservative, can be as high as 80 per cent in some preparations.

Lotions are dilutions of the mother tincture, usually by about 1:10 tincture:water, but up to about 1:50. They can be applied externally as often as desired to control suppuration and promote healing. When applied direct to the skin they may also have a drying effect. When added to gauze, as a dressing for a wound, the gauze should not be allowed to dry out. Lotion can be re-applied to the outside of a dressing before it dries, so the dressing may need to be changed less often.

Potencies are higher dilutions of the mother tincture than are lotions, and are given internally. The dilutions used by homeopaths are very high by allopathic standards, but homeopaths maintain that this very dilution produces a medicinal action not yet properly researched.

Normally, 1 part of mother tincture is added to 9 parts water, and shaken rhythmically. This is known as a 1x (decimal) dilution, or 1 part in 10. One part of this is then taken and added to another 9 parts water, and again shaken, to give a 2x dilution, or 1 part in 100. Similarly, a 3x dilution is 1 part in 1000, and a 6x is 1 part per million. These dilutions, also known as **potencies**, can be repeated a lot of times; the higher the dilution, the higher the potency number.

Dilutions are also made on a centesimal scale, or 1 part in 100, yielding 1c, 2c, and so on. A 6c potency, commonly recommended in this book, is a dilution of 1 in 10 followed by 12 zeroes. A 12c potency, often used by homeopaths, is a dilution of 1 in 10 followed by 24 zeroes, very close to the point at which there is none of the original substance remaining in a normal dose of about 6 drops. Yet the medicine still works, and many notable cures have been obtained at these dilutions.

The shaking procedure is known as **succussion,** and is regarded by homeopaths as an essential part of the dilution stage. Together, the dilution and succussion process is known as **potentization,** and can be repeated many thousands of times in the preparation of the medicines.

Although medicines for domestic use are not normally used above 6c and 12c, much higher potencies can be obtained from homeopaths for more specialized treatment. A number of 30c potencies, recommended for protection against infectious diseases such as influenza and measles, for example, are included in this book, and can be obtained from any homeopathic practitioner or homeopathic dispensary. Higher potencies are best obtained from a homeopath after consultation.

Mention should also be made of the tissue salts, which are homeopathic preparations of the twelve main mineral salts found in the body. These are also called cell salts and biochemic salts, and are widely available as homeopathic pilules in a 6x potency through health food shops and homeopathic pharmacies. Their use now has extended for over a century since their development by Dr. William Schuessler in Europe, and they are a valuable addition to any domestic homeopathic kit.

SAFETY

The safety of a wide variety of homeopathic medicines has been checked by government authorities. You would need to drink about five liters of a homeopathic medicine above 3x before you would begin to poison yourself. Anyone trying this would be unconscious from the alcohol, used as the preservative, before they approached a toxic dose. Since domestic doses are normally about 6 drops, a further safety factor is built in.

As a result, homeopathic medicines are particularly useful for home treatments. They are of good use in a wide range of disorders—for infants, children, women, men and the elderly. Therefore it is in the service of humanity that this book is presented.

PART ONE

Homeopathy: How Does It Work?

1

Explaining Homeopathy

The rising profile of homeopathy has produced something of a dilemma in the world of medicine: does it work or doesn't it? The decision bites deep: if homeopathic medicine is nothing but fraud, quackery and placebo, as many of its opponents would maintain, then a large number of competently trained homeopaths and doctors, together with countless thousands of dedicated lay practitioners, have been led up the medical garden path. Their millions of patients, including many heads of state and prominent members of several of Europe's royal families, have fallen victim to the most successful medical hoax ever perpetrated. On the other hand, if homeopathic medicine is effective, then for the first time in more than a hundred years the Western world is on the verge of accepting an entirely new system of medicine. Unlike modern pharmaceutical drugs, homeopathic medicines are non-toxic and easily manufactured; they are also very cheap.

During its 170 years of existence, homeopathy has been the center of continual and often bitter medical controversy. It has been particularly opposed by orthodox medicine, otherwise known as allopathy. But recently, both research and patient support has grown at a rapid pace. Yet rather than being hailed as a possible new medical breakthrough to give better health for all, it has been ridiculed, ignored and systematically suppressed.

Clearly, something is wrong. The problem is that homeopathic medicines can be diluted to such extremes that it can be shown physically, chemically, and mathematically that there is nothing in the final dose but water. Obviously then, the objection goes, any medicinal effect is nothing but placebo, and the homeopaths are both frauds and charlatans.

Yet the origins of homeopathic medicine are both honorable and orthodox. It was developed in Germany by the research of Dr. Samuel Hahnemann (1755–1834), who as well as being an experienced orthodox physician was also a competent chemist, a good mineralogist and botanist, and an able translator of eight different languages. His research stemmed from a dissatisfaction with the standard medical practices of his time: routine bleedings, heroic purgings with cathartics, and administration of large doses of crude drugs. While translating into German the *Materia Medica* by William Cullen, a Scottish professor of medicine, he was struck by a hitherto unexplored medical observation, first mentioned by Hippocrates. Cullen had proposed that the notable success of cinchona (an extract of quinine bark) in the treatment of swamp fever was due to its value as a stomach tonic. Hahnemann disagreed, and in his research on the question decided to take a course of the cinchona extract himself. To his surprise, he developed a set of symptoms remarkably similar to those of the swamp fever it was used to treat. All the symptoms disappeared when he stopped taking it. Further administration to himself and his family always produced the same symptoms, varying only in degree.

This was a strange phenomenon, uncited in the medical literature of the day: a remedy that was effective in a particular disease would produce a similar set of symptoms in a healthy person, when given in sufficient doses. In searching for precedents for this effect, he established that the first mention made of it was in the writings of Hippocrates (460–377 BC), regarded by the orthodoxy as the father of modern medicine. Hippocrates had said that likes can be cured by likes: that vomiting may be stopped by being made to vomit, and any illness caused by one means can be treated successfully by a similar means.

THE LAW OF SIMILARS

From this Hahnemann produced the first axiom of homeopathy, *Similia Similibus Curentur*—Let Likes be Cured by Likes, otherwise known as the Law of Similars—and so began his life's work. By 1821 he had produced two major works: *The Organon of Rational Medicine*, embodying the principles of the homeopathic approach to medicine, and his *Materia Medica Pura*, covering the effects of 64 medicines.

His approach to medicine represented a dramatic move away from the established method. Allopaths establish the existence of a particular disease, clarify its symptoms, and then test the effectiveness of various medicines on it, by the use of opposites. An illness accompanied by fever and diarrhea, for example, would call for the combined use of medicines that are anti-febrile and others that normally constipate, and so, in a crude way, a total balance would be found by using a number of appropriate medicines together.

Homeopaths tried the opposite approach: first test a substance for medicinal use, they said, by giving it to healthy volunteers, and carefully noting the symptoms it produces. This is known as a "proving." Once the symptom picture has been fully developed over a number of human trials, then the remedy can be assessed for usefulness against diseases with a similar set of symptoms. A substance that produces a bizarre set of symptoms such as bright red orifices and blue–green discharges, for example, will have little use in homeopathic clinical practice because symptoms of this type are rarely met. However a substance that produces a runny nose, watery, red eyes and repeated sneezing would be of great value in the treatment of hay fever. The common onion produces just those symptoms (as countless cooks can guarantee) and by use of the above trial system the onion has now achieved an established place in homeopathic therapeutics.

In essence, allopathic medicine embodies the law of opposites, homeopathic medicine the law of similars.

POTENTIZATION

At first the homeopathic approach to medicine seems contradictory. Surely experience tells us that exposing hay fever sufferers to large doses of onion would just add insult to injury, and make them worse rather than better. The homeopaths would agree, but with two provisos.

First, the symptoms must match closely before onion will have a therapeutic effect; this is embodied in their Law of the Single Remedy, which states that the most effective result will come from the most similar remedy, given in single doses. Then after the initial aggravation of symptoms dies down, the hay fever will be noticeably better.

Second, if the initial doses of onion are sufficiently diluted, there will be very little aggravation at all before improvement sets in. In fact, the homeopaths see dilution to infinitesimal degrees as a necessary part of the preparation of their medicines. It is embodied in the other important axiom for treatment: the Law of the Minimal Dose. This states that the most effective dose for a disorder is the minimum amount necessary to produce a response. Give one dose only of the diluted substance, the homeopaths say, and then wait for a favorable reaction. Having produced the desired improvement, give a second dose only when improvement stops.

It is this dilution of homeopathic medicines that has been the greatest obstacle to their more universal acceptance. The process is known as potentization, and involves a sequence of progressive dilution and a rhythmic shaking, termed succussion. In the normal case, 1 part of the source substance is added to 9 parts of water and shaken rhythmically. This is known as a 1x (decimal) dilution, or 1 part in 10 (also written as 10^{-1}). One part of this is then taken and added to another 9 parts of water, and again succussed, to give a 2x dilution, or 1 part in 100 (10^{-2}). Similarly, a 3x dilution is 1 part in 1000 (10^{-3}). These dilutions, also known as potencies, can be repeated a large number of times.

Dilutions are also made on a centesimal scale, or 1 part in 100, yielding 1c, 2c and so on. It needs only a little mental arithmetic to appreciate that a dilution procedure of this type (either decimal or centesimal) rapidly disperses the original substance. Table 1 gives a summary of the potencies, and their corresponding dilutions.

THE AVOGADRO LIMIT
In practice, a convenient classification of the dilutions is usually used.
- Low potencies: 1x–30x, or 1c–15c.
- Medium potencies: 30c–200c.
- High potencies: above 200c.

	DECIMAL SCALE	CENTESIMAL SCALE	CONCENTRATION
Table 1 Comparison of homeo-pathic potencies	1x	1c	10^{-1}
	2x	2c	10^{-2}
	3x	3c	10^{-3}
	4x	6c	10^{-4}
	6x	12c	10^{-6}
	12x	15c	10^{-12}
	24x	30c	10^{-24}
	30x	200c	10^{-24}
		1,000c (IM)	10^{-30}
		10,000c (IOM)	10^{-60}
		100,000c (CM)	10^{-400}
		1,000,000c (MM)	10^{-2000}
			$10^{-20,000}$
			$10^{-200,000}$
			$10^{-2,000,000}$

You will notice that the low potencies have been diluted least, and may still contain significant amounts of the source drug. But at a dose of 12c or 24x what is known as the Avogadro limit is reached, and at this concentration it is unlikely that even a single molecule of the original drug is still present in one liter of the preparation. Yet the Avogadro limit occurs in the low potency range and homeopaths maintain that, contrary to expectations, the power of the medicine increases as the potency increases.

So there is very little doubt that many patients treated with high potencies receive nothing but water.

Figure 1

The homeopathic dilutions

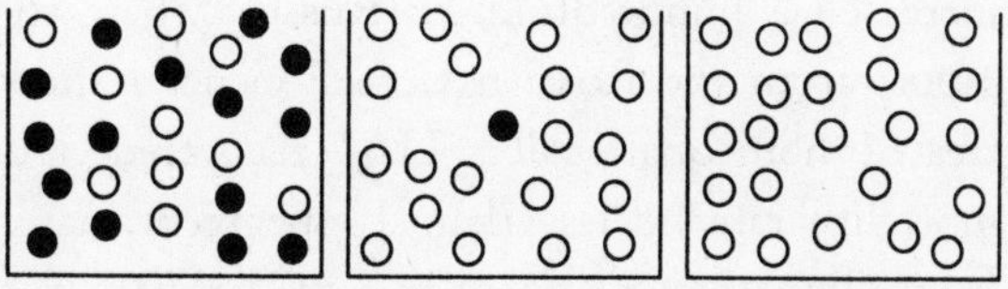

BELOW 24X	24X	ABOVE 24X
Many molecules of course drug per liter	Perhaps 1 molecule per liter	Low probability of even 1 molecule per liter

While the toxicity of such medicines is obviously very low, their efficacy has been seriously questioned, as dilutions above 12c can be dismissed on pharmacological grounds as completely inert. Yet potencies in the medium to high dilution range are the normal working area of homeopathy, and many striking cures have been claimed using them. The first and obvious response by allopaths is to claim that the action in successful cases is purely placebo, and the medicine is useful only to the suggestible and the gullible. Not so, maintain the homeopaths, who claim cures on infants, animals, unconscious patients, those with infectious diseases, and those with deep-seated, chronic disorders. In addition, the clinical trials are impressive. So the medical plot thickens.

CLINICAL TRIALS

The early homeopaths were all trained allopaths and, once having been convinced of the effectiveness of homeopathic medicines, felt no need to prove anything to anybody. After all, they had the training to use whatever medicine they considered appropriate for their patients. It was also expedient for them to make as little noise as possible about their use of a medical system that was already regarded as suspect within their own ranks. In any case, most of their research time was spent on provings, in order to expand the number of known and useful medicines, and very little on clinical trials.

As a result, it took an event of considerable magnitude to bring homeopathy out into the open, and the European cholera epidemic of 1832, two years before Hahnemann's death, was the occasion. By all accounts the homeopaths had a far higher recovery rate than the allopaths; it is said that in Paris the price of the homeopathic medicine for cholera increased a hundredfold. In Russia (where the epidemic originated), the report from the Russian Consul-General showed that of the 1270 cases treated homeopathically, 1162 recovered and only 108 died, giving a mortality rate of less than 10 per cent. By contrast, the mortality rate from allopathic treatment was 60 to 70 per cent.[1]

Following the homeopathic success in this epidemic medical interest in homeopathy increased at a rapid rate, and by the time of the next European cholera epidemic in 1854 the London Homoeopathic Hospital was already established. Its facilities were turned over entirely to the treatment of cholera victims, and the results were impressive. The homeopathic death rate was 16.4 per cent, compared to the allopathic death rate of 51.8 per cent. Similar successful figures were reluctantly reported by a number of other countries.[2] In Britain detailed returns had to be made by all hospitals and practitioners as to treatment and results in cholera, and the totals published by the British Medical Council in their *Blue Book of Statistics*. However, the figures from the Homoeopathic Hospital were deliberately omitted, and were only produced after considerable protest. The official reason for the omission was that inclusion of the homeopathic figures[2] "would give an unjustifiable sanction to an empirical practice, alike opposed to the maintenance of truth and the progress of science."

This prejudiced and bigoted reaction to the success of homeopathic medicine is typical of the problem that has plagued the advance of science for many centuries. Orthodox medicine, in particular, is well known for its poor track record in meeting innovative change and research breakthroughs with the proper degree of scientific detachment and quiet encouragement. Even within their own ranks some of the greatest of innovators, such as Lister, Jenner and Harvey, suffered ridicule and professional ostracism over discoveries that later became mainstays of medical practice. In reaction to homeopathic successes, the modern orthodox call has been for more clinical trials. Give us controlled trials, many allopaths have said, and if successful, we will accept the medicine.

Since that time, a number of clinical trials have been run, but many of them with poor controls. Some of the better-run trials are summarized here briefly. Those looking for a more complete list could do no better than the excellent review of Scofield.[3]

Mustard gas

The best controlled of the early clinical trials was conducted jointly in London and Glasgow during the Second World War, to find a method of prevention and treatment of mustard-gas burns. Mustard gas in the 6c potency, given as a preventative, reduced the incidence of deep and medium burns significantly. The remedies Rhus tox and Kali bich also gave statistically significant results in treatment.[4]

Rheumatoid arthritis

More recent trials were conducted in 1978 at the Glasgow Homoeopathic Hospital, now emerging as a stronghold of homeopathic research. Gibson and co-workers conducted a double-blind comparison of a range of homeopathic remedies in the treatment of rheumatoid arthritis (matched against the individual symptom pictures), and compared the patients' responses to those of salicylates and placebo. They showed that the patients who received homeopathic remedies responded statistically better than those who received salicylates; moreover, 42 per cent of the homeopathic group were able to discontinue all other treatment during the year.[5]

Objections to the method of trial led to a more rigidly designed trial in 1980, where patients were given either a homeopathic medicine or a placebo, but were allowed to continue with their orthodox anti-inflammatory drugs. The homeopathic group showed significant improvement as judged by a number of tests, as compared to the patients who received placebo. It was noted that homeopathy was a safer and no less effective alternative to present-day second-line drugs in the treatment of rheumatoid arthritis.[6]

HOMEOPATHIC REMEDIES NOT PLACEBO—THE CRACK WIDENS

One of the most recent clinical trials, and certainly the most tightly controlled to date, was conducted in 1986 at the Glasgow Homoeopathic Hospital by David Taylor Reilly, an allopath by training. The claim that homeopathic medicines are placebo was tested in a randomized, double-blind, placebo-controlled trial. In statistical terms, this is about as tough a trial as can be set up.

The effects of a homeopathic preparation of mixed grass pollens (30c potency, no molecules of the original pollen remaining) were compared with those of a placebo in a total of 144 patients with active hay fever. The homeopathically treated patients showed a statistically significant reduction in symptoms as assessed by both patient and physician. No evidence emerged to support the idea that placebo action explains the clinical response to homeopathic remedies.[7]

The publishing of Reilly's results in the *Lancet*, arguably the most prestigious medical journal in the world, indicates the current depth of penetration of homeopathic medicine into the allopathic world. The controversy it produced indicated the degree of crystallization of the collective allopathic brain. Here at last was proof positive in the much upheld double-blind trial, yet the collective reaction was less than positive. Although some of the more far-sighted of the correspondents suggested the possibility that a new chemistry and a new physics had been born, the reliance on pharmacology in the allopathic way of thinking showed its dominance. Reactions to drugs are caused by molecules of drug substances interacting with various body components, the thinking goes, and if there are no drug molecules in a medicine then there is no reaction aside from placebo effects. The experiment was simply testing one placebo against another. The fact that statistical significance was obtained for one of the "placebos" was apparently deemed of no consequence, and indicates that the issue may not be a scientific issue at all, but more an economic and emotional one.

PHARMACOLOGICAL SUPPORT

Logically, one of the first areas to investigate for support (or the lack of it) in homeopathy is the area of pharmacology, or drug action. And, contrary to expectations, some surprising support is appearing.

Ask a pharmacologist about the biological effect of very low concentrations of common substances on living organisms and the answer will be that there is typically very little or zero response. Ask for some theoretical backup, and in short order you will find yourself confronted by one of the pharmacological tools of the trade, the Dose–Response curve. In brief, the curve illustrates one of the rules of thumb in drug use: that an increased dose of drug will give an increased effect, while a lowered dose of a drug will give a reduced effect, and a very low dose will give no effect at all.

A glance at the curve in Figure 2 will show that the pharmacologically recommended dose of a drug lies in the area of the ED_{50}, the dose that produces 50 per cent of the total or maximum effect. The homeopathic area of interest, on the other hand, lies at the very start of the curve, in the area of the so-called threshold dose.

The area of the threshold dose is usually avoided in standard pharmacological drug testing, for two reasons. The first is that the threshold dose lies some distance from the area of the ED_{50}, so investigating this area for drug reaction is basically a waste of time. But the other reason is far more interesting. The threshold dose is an area where paradoxical and contradictory results are obtained, not easily explained in conventional terms. Again, the easy answer is to simply avoid it in experimentation. But the bottom line is that for many years the pharmacologists have known of the strange results obtained in the threshold

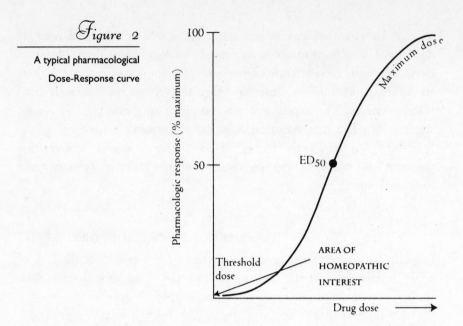

Figure 2

A typical pharmacological
Dose-Response curve

Pharmacologic response (% maximum)

100

50 — ED$_{50}$

Maximum dose

Threshold
dose

AREA OF
HOMEOPATHIC
INTEREST

Drug dose ⟶

dose area, but have simply chosen to ignore them. In doing so, they have unwittingly withdrawn orthodox support for an entirely different field of medicine.

It is interesting that one of the very earliest laws of pharmacology, known as the Arndt–Schulz Law, had already expressed the homeopathic effect. Formulated by Arndt in 1888, and restated by Hueppe a few years later, the law set the groundwork for what should have been a side-by-side development of allopathic and homeopathic medicine in the following century. It states: *For every substance, small doses stimulate, moderate doses inhibit, large doses kill.*

Allopathic medicine, with its emphasis on moderate drug doses, works in the inhibitory part of the scale. The result is seen in the typically inhibitory medicines produced: antihistamines, antibiotics, antacids, cough suppressants and so on, laying the basis for the so-called "suppressant" effect of drugs.

Homeopathic medicine, on the other hand, begins at the stimulatory end of the curve, and moves to the left, into the smaller and smaller dose range. Its emphasis is on the stimulation of the body's natural balancing mechanisms, as seen in its philosophy of the natural regeneration of the body through rebuilding of vitality, a concept also in close agreement with naturopathic thought.

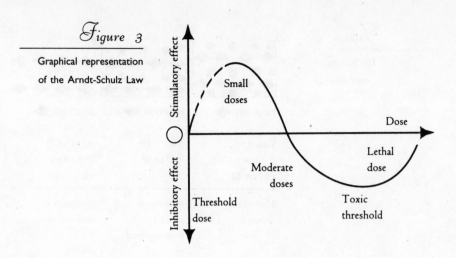

Figure 3

Graphical representation
of the Arndt-Schulz Law

The pioneering work of Dr William Boyd in the early 1940s[8] bound the worlds of homeopathy and Arndt–Schulz together with a series of tightly controlled experiments, and set the stage for work much later on as to how homeopathic medicine may work. Boyd worked with the enzyme malt diastase, which was already known to be inhibited by crude doses of the salt mercuric chloride, and measured its speed in the hydrolysis of starch. He also used a number of homeopathically prepared dilutions of mercuric chloride, including a batch at 61x, where there was no likelihood of any of the original salt remaining—it was pure water. He additionally worked with distilled water as a control. He showed that crude doses of mercuric chloride inhibited diastase activity, as was already well known, and that distilled water had no effect. But he also showed, with statistically significant results, that *mercuric chloride 61x* accelerated diastase activity.

Now this experiment had a number of ramifications, besides supporting the Arndt–Schulz Law. If there was no mercuric chloride in the 61x potency, the malt diastase should have reacted the same as distilled water. If, on the other hand, there was a contamination of mercuric chloride somehow in the test doses, then the activity of the diastase enzyme should have decreased. Instead it did neither, but increased. From the laboratory point of view, homeopathic medicines not only had been shown to work according to the Arndt–Schulz Law, but had been shown to affect enzyme action.

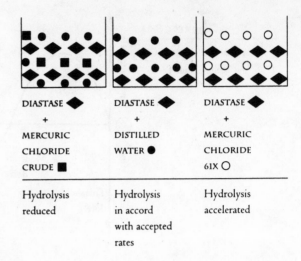

Figure 4

The activity of malt diastase

DIASTASE ◆	DIASTASE ◆	DIASTASE ◆
+	+	+
MERCURIC	DISTILLED	MERCURIC
CHLORIDE	WATER ●	CHLORIDE
CRUDE ■		61X ○
Hydrolysis reduced	Hydrolysis in accord with accepted rates	Hydrolysis accelerated

HORMESIS: THE NEW BREAKTHROUGH

Look up the Arndt–Schulz Law in a modern textbook of pharmacology and you will be lucky if you find it mentioned, let alone discussed. It died out of the textbooks as allopathic interest moved further into the inhibitory part of the Arndt–Schulz curve, and as the pharmacological Dose–Response curve avoided the area of the threshold dose. It appeared that, for all its promising origins, theoretical support for homeopathy had died a natural death.

Recently, however, further support for homeopathic medicine has come from a most unlikely direction: the field of toxicology, or the action of poisons. Beginning in 1960, data began to accumulate that poisonous substances were having two effects on living organisms.[9] At high doses they inhibited metabolism and ultimately caused death, as was well known. But at low doses they exerted a stimulating effect, a response totally unexpected and not explainable by current medical science. Recently the trickle turned to a torrent, as toxicologists have turned to examine the new phenomenon of hormesis, the name given to the stimulatory effect of low levels of usually poisonous substances.[10–15] The Arndt–Schulz Law has not died: it has simply resurfaced with a new name.

The research results are incomplete, but the trend is inescapable. Evidence from experiments, both human and animal, shows hormesis as an effect occurring in all biological domains tested, with growing research support. It demonstrates that all substances (including pesticides and carcinogens) that show an inhibitory effect at high concentrations, have a stimulatory effect at low concentrations.

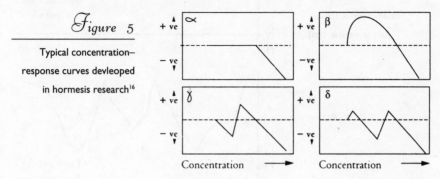

Figure 5

Typical concentration–
response curves devleoped
in hormesis research[16]

In Figure 5 the alpha (α) curve is the most expected pattern, and is assumed to describe the actions of drugs in humans as the concentration moves from low concentrations to progressively more inhibitory ones. This curve is a tentative one, and is assigned to those drugs that have not yet been fully tested for a stimulatory response.

The beta (β) curve was the most frequently observed pattern, and accounted for the human reactions to the bulk of the drugs tested. It shows a typical curve as predicted by the Arndt–Schulz Law, but (understandably) was not tested in toxic and lethal dose ranges.

The two other curves, the gamma (γ) and delta (δ) forms, were recorded where data was available for biological response at lower dose ranges. However, data points for these ranges are generally less available, so the validity of these curves is unknown until further data is available.

Homeopathic research has consistently produced results showing the basic curve structure of hormesis and the Arndt–Schulz Law. But the research goes further: as the drug substance is progressively diluted, the biological reaction alternates between stimulation and inhibition, as given by the hormesis gamma and delta curves. This periodic behavior is called *rhythmicity* by homeopaths, and represents one of the several great unexplained phenomena in homeopathic action. But one factor has been established: as the dilutions become extreme and the concentration of the source drug approaches zero, the biological reaction will also fade out unless the diluted solution is succussed in accord with traditional homeopathic practice.

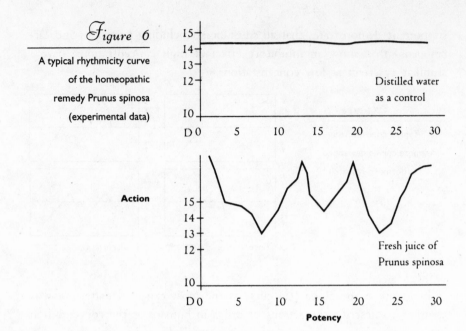

Figure 6

A typical rhythmicity curve
of the homeopathic
remedy Prunus spinosa
(experimental data)

15
14
13
12
10

D 0   5   10   15   20   25   30

Distilled water
as a control

Action

15
14
13
12
10

D 0   5   10   15   20   25   30

Potency

Fresh juice of
Prunus spinosa

HOW DOES HOMEOPATHY WORK?

Central to the issue of medical acceptance of homeopathy is the clarification of its mechanism of action. In particular, is there a model that adequately explains its clinical effectiveness and the successes of the trials?

In the development of a workable model, the research thinking has gone something like this: given that homeopathic medicine is effective even when it can be shown that there is no likelihood of any molecules being left in a particular dose (due to dilution), then the effect of the dose must lie with the water molecules themselves, since that is all that is left. Water itself can be assumed to have no effect in this case, since the dose is small, and the effect would always be the same. The answer must lie within the water molecules, and the only real possibility is in the type of energy that the molecule has stored.

Energy storage within molecules in biological systems lies within the realm of biophysics rather than biochemistry. Biophysics is a new field, having become established only within the last twenty years or so. It is not yet included in medical curricula in universities to any great extent, and is only now beginning to make its mark in the biological sciences. Small wonder, therefore, that the established medical world knows little of its existence, or the promise it holds in explaining the action of the medicines of energy, such as homeopathy, acupuncture, psychic and spirit healing and radionics.

ENERGY STORAGE

Molecules such as water can store energy in four different ways—as motion, spin, vibration and electronic excitation. Some storage modes can store more energy than others, and we will start at the lowest, least energetic mode, which is kinetic energy, or energy of motion. A molecule stores kinetic energy by virtue of its speed. It is this storage in gases and liquids that causes pressure (such as air pressure) by the continual collision of the molecules with surfaces like our skin, and also causes the bulk of chemical reactions to occur. At room temperature, the energy that these molecules contain is low, compared with other states. It is unlikely to be associated with homeopathic medicine's effects, since the energy is constantly altered by collision, and so any energy stored is quickly degraded.

SPIN AND MICROWAVE COOKING

Spin energy is found in gases and liquids, but not in solids, where the stronger attractions between molecules prevents rotation. It is also not found in water until it reaches about 108°F (42°C), a factor of considerable importance to living organisms, composed as they are of up to 90 per cent water, with humans being about 40 per cent. Heating water to about 108°F causes sufficient disruption of the molecular attraction between molecules to allow spin to occur, and that's precisely the temperature at which humans start to die. Life processes in general seem to keep a safe distance from the temperature band of 108–113°F.

Spin energy in molecules corresponds to microwave radiation, which is one reason why this radiation is lethal. It is also an indication of the potential power of energy storage in this mode—strong enough to cook food. But it is unlikely to be the source of action of homeopathic medicine, since at room temperature the spin storage state in water has not become active.

Figure 7

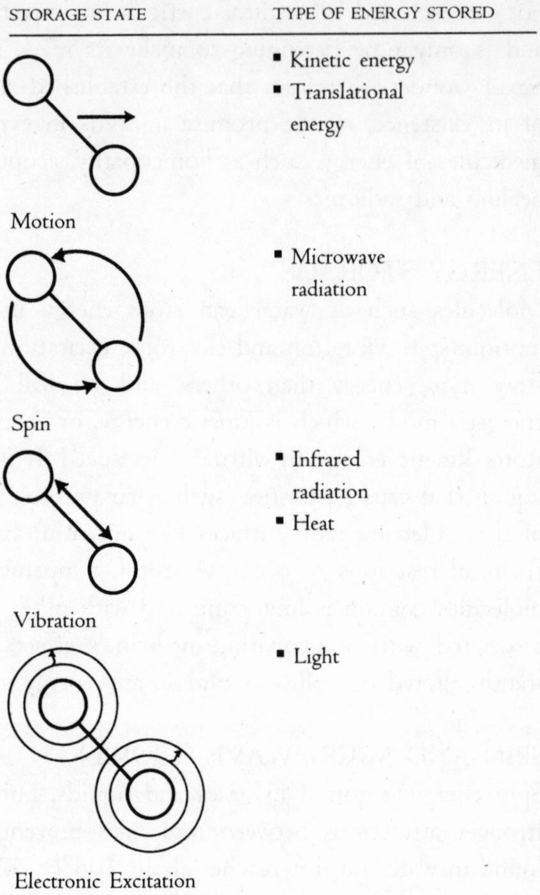

STORAGE STATE	TYPE OF ENERGY STORED

Energy storage in molecules

Motion
- Kinetic energy
- Translational energy

Spin
- Microwave radiation

Vibration
- Infrared radiation
- Heat

Electronic Excitation
- Light

ELECTRONIC EXCITATION

At the top end of the scale is electronic excitation, which is the stuff powering lasers, of great strength and intensity. Excite the electrons circling the component molecules up into higher orbits and energy is stored. Drop them down together, and a pulse of light is given out. It may be of sufficient strength and power to burn a hole through a razor blade, cut tissue in surgery, or stop an army tank—it depends on what molecules are used, and how strongly the electrons are excited. Again, it is unlikely to be the source of action of homeopathic medicine, because the excited electrons are unstable, and will decay to their previous state in a matter of fractions of a second.

VIBRATORY STORAGE

Standing midway between the cooking power of microwave and the destructive power of lasers is vibratory energy. Although it has an accepted place in physics as a means of storing energy, it has had a chequered career in medical science because of its association with trance mediums, psychic phenomena and extrasensory perception. Vibratory energy can be found in molecules throughout all three states of matter—solid, liquid and gas. It is responsible for phenomena such as the expansion of metals when heated, and the transfer of heat by conduction. Vibratory motion of a molecule increases when the molecule absorbs energy, and this vibratory energy can be re-radiated at a later time, usually in the infrared part of the spectrum, where heat is also found.

It is in the *storage* of vibratory energy in water molecules during the succussion process that homeopathic medicine places many of its hopes for a scientific explanation of its action. It is proposed that during the collision process, vibratory energy is exchanged between the source drug and the water, and that the water is left with a vibratory imprint of the drug. Further succussion makes the imprint deeper, which explains why the medicines are regarded as acting more strongly as the dilution increases. Furthermore it is not just energy that is being stored, it is proposed, but information, differing from one remedy to another depending on the source substance used, with every substance leaving a different vibratory signature in the water molecule. In this way homeopathic medicine is seen as carrying information into the body when it is taken in dose form, perhaps as biological instructions.

If water molecules were dissociated from each other (moving freely in all directions) at room temperature, any vibratory energy stored would quickly degrade. But at 77° (25°C) about 70 per cent of water molecules are incorporated into a stable, hexagonal, lattice structure, capable of storing a considerable amount of vibratory energy before it breaks up. However, storage of vibratory energy causes structural changes, because any molecule that absorbs energy will always change its shape. So a convenient way of telling if this particular model was possible was to examine homeopathic water for structural changes.

A number of workers over the years have shown that both high and low potency homeopathic medicines show structural changes in the water they contain. It was additionally shown that in order for the structural changes to occur, two things must happen. First, there must be a source drug to begin with: that is, you can't make a homeopathic medicine from water alone. Second, you must succuss the remedy as it is diluted stepwise, in the rhythmic shaking manner used by the homeopaths for many years. Only when these two processes are included will structural changes show.

BENVENISTE—CHAMPION OR CHARLATAN?

In one of the stranger episodes in the recorded history of scientific publishing, the prestigious British research journal *Nature* recently published experimental results which the editors say they consider utterly impossible. The paper, "Human Basophil Degranulation Triggered by Very Dilute Antiserum Against IgE"[17], and the conclusions it proposes, has stirred up substantial controversy in the medical community.

The main players in the experiment were an eminent French medical researcher, Professor Benveniste, a special type of white blood cell known as a basophil, and an antibody, IgE. When basophils are normally exposed to this antibody, their chemistry and internal structure change, in a way that is easily checked by staining techniques. But what Benveniste and his colleagues found was that the changes occurred even when the antibody was used up to the 120x potency, a dilution at which it is mathematically impossible for even one molecule of the antibody to remain.

The results also showed the familiar rhythmic changes in basophil reactions as the potencies increased, a factor still unexplained even by homeopaths. The deputy editor of *Nature* remarked that two centuries of observation and rational thinking about biology will have to be abandoned if the results stand, because they cannot be explained by existing physical laws.

The 13-member international research team headed by Professor Benveniste conducted their experiments after being challenged by two eminent French homeopaths to disprove homeopathy. To settle the question once and for all, they conducted a sensitive, tightly controlled experiment at the University of South Paris, where Professor Benveniste is a research director. "That was how it all started," he said. "They challenged us to prove them wrong, and we couldn't." Instead, the experiment showed strong support for homeopathy.

The furor surrounding this experiment has produced some unique reactions within the scientific community, and highlights an important question: how should the scientific establishment deal with findings that challenge the very roots of established thought? *Nature* had its own answer: it sent a fraud squad comprising one of its editors, a professional magician

Table 2

Structural changes in high and low potency homeopathic medicines[18]

WORKERS	PREPARATION	MEASURED	FINDINGS
Wurmser and Loch, 1948	Several substances from 24x to 30x	Intensity and wavelength of light by photoelectric cell	Measurable changes for several substances
Gay and Boiron, 1951-3	Distilled water alone, and with several additions of sodium chloride 27c	Dielectric constant	Could select the single bottle with sodium chloride 27c from 99 control bottles
Boericke and Smith, 1963	12x dilution of sulphur with and without succussion	Solvent structure by nuclear magnetic resonance spectrum	Structural change in solvent as the potency is increased with succussion; no change in control
Stephenson and Brucato, 1966	Distilled water, mercuric chloride 1x to 33x	Dielectric constant For controls, the dielectric constant varied from 5.6 to 6.05. For homeopathic dilutions, it varied from 2.80 to 4.40	
Young, 1975	Sulphur from 5x to 30x, with controls	Solvent structure by nuclear magnetic resonance spectrum	Measurable changes in spectra at each dilution and succussion. No changes for solutions without succussion or without sulphur

and an investigator of scientific frauds from the USA to Benveniste's laboratories. Over a period of a week they criticized shortcomings in experimental design, studied the laboratory records and interrogated the researchers. Finally, they failed to replicate the results in a double-blind trial, and declared the experiments "a delusion." Professor Benveniste, not unexpectedly, considered the investigation a witch hunt and an outrage. "I welcome any explanation for our findings on homeopathy," he said, "but not this kind of rubbish."

NEW FINDINGS—A RECENT SURVEY OF CLINICAL TRIALS

As a useful summary of all published trials, a recent paper in the *British Medical Journal* reviewed the evidence of 107 homeopathic trials from 96 published reports.[19] Most of the trials were considered to be of poor quality; however, there were exceptions. The best trials were those by Grecho and by Reilly. Reilly's trial was to test whether homeopathic medicines were placebo, and came out in favor of the medicine being therapeutically active. The Grecho trial was specialized, and some would argue out of the realm of homeopathy: it looked at recovery of bowel movements after surgery and gave a negative result.

Overall the results of all trials showed a positive trend, regardless of the quality of the trial or the prescribing system used. Of the 105 trials with interpretable results, 81 trials indicated positive results using homeopathic remedies, while in 24 no positive effects were found.
A more interesting, and perhaps more useful, result can be drawn from looking at the most recent trials, which were also the most tightly controlled. Of these trials, nine showed a positive result in favour of homeopathy being therapeutically valid, and two gave negative findings.

The review concluded that the evidence from clinical trials was positive but not sufficient to draw definitive conclusions, and recommended more well-conducted trials. Nevertheless the homeopaths of the world can now be reassured that what we always knew to be true is at last starting to appear in the research: that homeopathy works.

HOMEOPATHY AROUND THE WORLD

Homeopathy is achieving increasing support and acceptance worldwide. Often it is being included as part of the global acceptance of natural medicine, but one fact stands out: there has been a substantial integration of homeopathy into the education and health-care systems of a number of countries. Figures worldwide are difficult to find, but the following items of information will help to set a global picture.

BELGIUM
All natural therapy practitioners are registered with a central medical council. One person in every four visits a natural therapist. Homeopathy is the most popular treatment.[20]

DENMARK
There are about 2000 registered natural therapists, including homeopaths. About one in 10 of the population go to them.[21]

FRANCE
In France 20,000 pharmacies sell homeopathic remedies, and many faculties of pharmacy award postgraduate diplomas in homeopathy. One quarter of all French doctors have prescribed homeopathic medicines. Acupuncture and homeopathy are taught in some university medical faculties. One in six patients is given homeopathic treatments.[22,23]

THE NETHERLANDS
The integration of orthodox and alternative medicines is encouraged by the government. Training in natural therapies is restricted to university-trained doctors.[24]

INDIA
The government directly supports and funds many of the 120 homeopathic medical colleges and research establishments in India. There are now 125,000 trained and registered degree-level homeopaths practicing throughout the country. There are over 2000 dispensaries and over 100 homeopathic hospitals, all government-funded. There is also a government-funded National Institute of Homeopathy in Calcutta. The president of India has an honorary homeopathic physician.[25]

SOUTH AFRICA
Education for naturopathy, homeopathy and herbalism is currently available at government-funded tertiary institutions.[26]

USA

It appears that in the United States there is now an enormous swing to alternative medicine. A recent report showed that more than one in three Americans had used alternative medicines at least once in 1990. Furthermore, the study found that patients made more than 425 million visits to alternative practitioners that year, in contrast to 388 million visits to family doctors and other primary care physicians. Among the 16 systems examined were chiropratic, vitamin therapy, massage, acupuncture, homeopathy, herbal medicine and spiritual healing. Affluent and well-educated 25–49-year-olds—the nation's most influential consumer group—were found to be most likely to try alternative health care.[27]

Although much of the modern development of homeopathy occurred in America because of the efforts of pioneers there such as James Tyler Kent and Constantine Hering, homeopathy in America has been largely suppressed. Now for the first time in many decades a conventional American medical school is running a course in homeopathic medicine. The first training program is now being offered at Arizona State University Medical School, and includes continuing medical education credits for practicing allopaths. Other courses, including weekend seminars, are pending approval. The two-year course will be followed by one year of clinical training.

UNITED KINGDOM

About one person in eight goes to a natural therapist. British law puts no restriction on natural therapists, who may take referrals from doctors. Homeopathy is practiced under the National Health Service, and has a wide level of acceptance. All homeopathic medicines prescribed by a doctor are available under the National Health Service; many doctors practice homeopathy and many pharmacists stock homeopathic medicines. The Queen and other members of the royal family have an appointed honorary homeopathic physician.[28-30]

A recent article published in the British medical journal *Doctor* looked at a survey of GPs' attitudes toward homeopathy. It reflects the growing acceptance of the medicine on a worldwide scale:

■ 80 per cent of all doctors said they believed homeopathy to be effective;

■ 92 per cent of female GPs believed in the effectiveness of homeopathy;

■ 20 per cent of all doctors said that homeopathy can be more effective than conventional medicine;

■ 43 per cent of doctors were willing to refer patients to homeopaths.

Interestingly, only 11 per cent had any homeopathic training, but 79 per cent wanted homeopathy included in medical training.

AUSTRALIA

Certainly in Australia homeopathic medicines are gaining new levels of acceptance, due mainly to the recent Therapeutic Goods and Cosmetic Act. This act was put into place to ensure that medicines sold in Australia were at a world standard of quality, safety and efficacy. Although most homeopathic medicines are exempt from the Australian Register of Therapeutic Goods set up by the Health Department, some specific remedies have already been included on the register. They must comply with standards of quality and safety, and must also comply with the same legislation as all other medicines concerning standards of manufacture and labeling.

Qualified homeopaths now have government recognition as health-care professionals under recent legislation. While official registration as Medicare providers will be a long time coming (if it comes at all), it is safe to say that homeopathy is now established in Australia.

Notes

1 Bradford's Logic of Figures (1900), *from* Tyler, 'Homeopathic Drug Pictures', *Health Science*, 1978.

2 Tyler, 'Homeopathic Drug Pictures', *Health Science*, 1978.

3 Scofield, 'Homeopathy and Its Potential Role in Agriculture. A critical review,' *Biol. Ag. Hort*, 2: 1–50, 1984.

4 Scofield, ibid.

5 Scofield, ibid.

6 Scofield, ibid.

7 Reilly *et al*, 'Is Homeopathy a Placebo Response?' *Lancet*, 881–6, 18 October 1986.

8 Boyd, 'The Action of Microdoses of Mercuric Chloride on Malt Diastase', *Brit. Hom. J.*, 31: 1–28, 1941 and 32: 106–11, 1942.

9 Townsend and Luckey, 'Hormoligosis in Pharmacology', *JAMA*, 44, 7 May 1960.

10 Stebbings, 'Hormesis—The Stimulation of Growth by Low Levels of Inhibitors', *Sci. Tot. Environ.*, 22: 213–34, 1982.

11 Bond *et al*, 'Microdosimetric Concepts Applied to Hormesis', *Health Physics*, 52 (5): 659–61, 1987.

12 Furst *et al*, 'Hormetic Effects in Pharmacology', *Health Physics*, 52 (5): 527–30.

13 Sagan, 'What Is Hormesis and Why Haven't We Heard of It Before?', *Health Physics*, 52 (5): 521–5.

14 Calabrese *et al*, 'The Occurence of Chemically Induced Hormesis', *Health Physics*, 52 (5): 531–41.

15 Brisbin *et al*, 'Sigmoid Growth and the Assessment of Hormesis', *Health Physics*, 52 (5): 553–9.

16 Stebbings, op. cit.

17 Coulter, *Homeopathic Science and Human Medicine*, North Atlantic, 1980.

18 Devenas, Benveniste *et al*, 'Human Basophil Degranulation Triggered by Very Dilute Antiserum Against IgE', *Nature* 33: 816–30, June 1988.

19 Kleijnen *et al*, 'Clinical trials of homeopathy', *BMJ* 302: 316–23, 1991.

20 *The Times*, 23 November 1989.

21 *The Times*, op. cit.

22 *The Times*, op. cit.

23 *Pharmaceutical Journal*, 19 September 1987.

24 *The Times*, op. cit.

25 Goel, Ministry of Health and Family Welfare, *Traditional Medicines: The Indian Scenario*, American Botanical Council Classical Reprint Number 201.

26 *South African Government Gazette*, 1982.

27 *New Eng. J. Med* 328; 246–52, 1993.

28 *Lancet* 108, 15 January 1983.

29 *Pharmaceutical Journal*, 29 October 1988.

30 Steinbach, *Pharmaceutical Journal*, 385–7, 3 October 1981.

PART TWO

Treatments

2

How to Use Homeopathic Medicines

Remedies should be stored in a cool, dark place such as a cupboard or drawer, and away from strong-smelling perfumes and liniments. They should not be stored in the refrigerator, nor close to microwave ovens or computers. They should be taken under the tongue in a clean mouth, preferably about half an hour before meals. Avoid drinking coffee completely while taking homeopathic medicines (tea, however, is okay), and do not take after using toothpaste.

SELECTING THE REMEDY

If you are familiar with homeopathic prescribing, you will know that homeopaths can ask patients many curious questions, and may base their choice of the correct remedy on a number of different and apparently unrelated conditions. Symptoms such as being worse in a draught, or always better in humid weather or in the open air, can decisively indicate the correct choice of remedy.

The remedies listed in this book have been chosen for a number of reasons: they are well suited to the disorders found in the average home, they are safe and easy to use, and they have clear-cut symptoms.
To begin with, you may care to rely on the descriptions of the symptoms given for each disorder in this book. By using this alone,

you will become a prescriber of some competence. But you will soon become aware that these medicines work best by treating the patient as an individual and the body as a whole. At about this time you would find Part Two, "A Materia Medica of Common Remedies," useful, as each remedy there is summarized, showing its main pattern of symptoms.

It is the understanding of the pattern of symptoms in a remedy—what the homeopaths call a **symptom picture**—that is the key to prescribing. A remedy that closely matches in its symptom picture the symptoms of the patient is known in homeopathy as the **similimum**, the most similar remedy, and is the one to prescribe. In these cases, its action is dramatic and gratifying, and quickly repays the effort of prescribing correctly.

DOSE

How often you give a medicine will depend on the potency you use, the type of illness, and the age of the patient. As a general rule, low potencies of 6x, or 3c, to 12c are used for acute complaints, such as colds, attacks of vomiting, wounds, and so on. Medium potencies of 30c are used in more established conditions such as recurrent migraines or entrenched period pain. Higher potencies, of 200c and above, are used in deeper constitutional treatment, and are best left to experienced prescribers.

Many of the potencies mentioned in this book are for 6x and 6c; these are good, fast-acting potencies, well suited to the majority of domestic disorders. They are available in a variety of dose forms, including liquids, pilules, tablets and oral sprays.

A normal dose of any liquid is about 6 drops, usually taken under the tongue, but the remedy can be rubbed into the chest in cases where opening the mouth is difficult. For frequent dosing, such as with a child at night, put half a capful, or about 20 drops, in 1 cm of water in a glass, and give by clean eye dropper.

Generally, a dose is given every 2–3 hours during the day. It can also be given at night if the patient is awake.

Tablets are placed under the tongue and allowed to dissolve, or can be chewed if preferred. The usual dose is 2 tablets for adults, 1 for children.

Pilules are small, round tablets, often used in homeopathic kits because they can be packed into space-saving bottles. The usual dose is 4 pilules for an adult, 2 pilules for a child. Like tablets, they are placed under the tongue and allowed to dissolve, or can be chewed if preferred.

Oral sprays are a recent introduction to the homeopathic market, and have proved to be very convenient. The usual dose is 4 sprays for an adult, 2 for a child.

For the low potencies of 6x, or 3–12c, one dose generally can be given every few hours until the patient improves or until a change occurs. If there is no change after one or two weeks, especially in acute illnesses, the remedy has probably failed and a new remedy should be chosen. Higher potencies are given less often. As a general rule, the 30c potency is given once a day, to adults and children, for several days. It is used most often in longer term disorders, such as arthritis or constipation, although it is sometimes given once a day for several weeks. For entrenched conditions, the 200c potency may be given once a week or once a month. Higher potencies, such as 1M, are given about once a month for constitutional problems.

Infants and children respond more quickly to remedies than do adults, although their symptoms are also liable to change more quickly, so they need to be watched closely. Particularly in infants, the results from a single dose can show within hours—even minutes—so the remedy can sometimes be given less often, such as morning and evening.

REMEDY REACTIONS

After giving a well-chosen remedy for a number of doses, one of three things can happen.

■ The symptoms persist
If given for three to six doses in an acute illness, or for several weeks in a more long-standing illness, and there is no improvement, the remedy has failed. The similimum was not chosen. A new remedy should be selected.
■ The symptoms improve
The remedy has succeeded, and dosage should be stopped. Further dosage should begin only when improvement stops.

■ The symptoms aggravate (worsen)
The remedy may be correct, but is stimulating a response. Dosage should be stopped. A marked improvement can be expected when the aggravation subsides. Further dosage should begin only when improvement stops, usually at a higher potency than the first remedy. If the aggravation continues, professional advice should be sought.

Any illness that fails to improve after the administration of apparently correct remedies should always receive professional assessment.

3
First Aid

Abrasions and Lacerations

Abrasions are wounds where the surface layer of skin has been taken off. Deeper damage, especially involving underlying muscle, nerves and blood vessels, is a **laceration**; these wounds are typically torn and jagged, and are often badly pulped.

The first action needed is always to stop any bleeding. Elevation of the wound (holding it higher than the rest of the body) will always help. Clean the wound as far as possible: holding it under cold running water will substantially remove debris although embedded particles may need to be removed with forceps or tweezers. Large wounds may need pressure to bring the edges together, and usually require allopathic treatment (stitching). Wounds containing badly pulped tissue, or showing uncontrollable suppuration, should also receive allopathic treatment.

TREATMENT

The choice of lotion or ointment to apply depends on the nature of the wound. Homeopathic lotions are known as **tinctures**, and may be put directly on the wound, or on a piece of gauze (the gauze should be kept moist). They are useful when maximum penetration of a wound is necessary. It is rarely necessary to apply the tincture undiluted, as a dilution of about 1 in 10 parts water works just as well, and is more economical. Ointments are more greasy, and do not penetrate as well as tinctures, but they have the advantage of sealing the wound to some extent and so the wound may not require further covering.

■ For wounds oozing dark, (venous) blood.
Hamamelis tincture diluted 1 in 10, applied locally.
Internally Hamamelis 6c, every 3–4 hours.

■ *For wounds with bright red (arterial) blood.*
Calendula tincture 1 in 10, applied locally.
Internally Calendula 6c, every 3–4 hours.

■ If local inflammation (redness, heat, swelling and tenderness) sets in.
Hepar sulph 6c, every 3–4 hours.

■ *For wounds likely to suppurate.*
Equal parts of Hypericum and Calendula tincture (Hypercal) diluted 1 in 10, applied locally.
Internally Calendula 6c, every few hours.

■ For pain that is sharp, intense and shooting.
Hypericum 6c internally, every 3–4 hours, or whenever the pain returns.

Bites and Stings

Ledum and **Apis** given internally are useful generally for treating insect bites and stings, and most symptoms will yield rapidly using these two remedies alone.

Allergic reactions to insect bites should be treated differently: these appear as rapid and large swellings, beginning at the site of the sting and spreading out. If the sting is on the neck, if it causes breathing difficulty, or if the person has a known sensitivity to stings, allopathic advice should be sought immediately.

TREATMENT

■ Immediately.
Lemon juice applied locally is a good first-line treatment.

■ As a general treatment.
Ledum tincture 1 in 10 externally, followed by Urtica tincture 1 in 10 if Ledum does not cause improvement.

- For mosquito bites or insect stings that feel worse from warm applications, and better from cold applications.
  Ledum 6c every 3–4 hours.
- *For bee or wasp stings, that are bright red and swollen, painful, burning and itching and that become worse in heat.*
  Apis 6c, every 3–4 hours.
- For ant bites, with sudden rheumatic and gouty pains.
  Formica rufa 6c, every 1–2 hours.

- For pain, in extremely sensitive areas, especially when it is darting or shooting.
  Hypericum 6c, every 3–4 hours, or whenever pain returns.
- To reduce infection and promote healing.
  Calendula 6c, every 3–4 hours.
- For shock after stings, if the person is anxious and restless.
  Aconite 6c, every 3–4 hours.
- For itchy, blotchy skin, with burning and pain.
  Urtica 6c, every 3–4 hours.

ANIMAL, SPIDER AND REPTILE BITES

These bites are dangerous, particularly snake and spider bites. In these cases, the entire limb should be wrapped in compressive bandages such as crepe bandage or panty hose as soon as possible after the event to reduce fluid flow. The limb should then be immobilised, and allopathic treatment should immediately be found. It should also be noted that human bites can be extremely infectious.

TREATMENT

The following remedies can be used while allopathic advice is being sought.

- As a local treatment.
  Ledum tincture applied to the bite as a compress.
- For spider and snake bites that are purple and oozing thin, dark blood, while allopathic treatment is being sought.
  Lachesis 12c, every 30 minutes.

- As a general treatment.
  Ledum 6c given internally, every 3–4 hours.
- For spider and snake bites that cause burning and itching, with unsteadiness and exhaustion, while allopathic treatment is being sought.
  Carbolic acid 6c, every 30 minutes.

- For bites that are swollen and blackish-purple in color, with swollen lymph nodes.
  Tarentula 12c, every 3–4 hours.

- For shock, anxiety, restlessness, or fear of death.
  Aconite 6c, every 3–4 hours.

TICK BITES

Using tweezers, try to remove the tick whole, taking special care to ensure the head is not left behind. Alternatively, put a drop of kerosene or olive oil on the tick—this may make it fall off.

TREATMENT

- As a local application.
  Ledum tincture 1 in 10, applied to the bite.
- For tick bite in animals, with paralysis of the rear limbs.
  Lathyrus 30c can be obtained from a practitioner.

- As a general treatment.
  Ledum 6c internally, every 3–4 hours.
- In collapse due to tick poisoning, with a craving for fresh air.
  Carbo veg 6c, every 3–4 hours, while allopathic treatment is being sought.

Bruises and Blows

Injuries of this type are usually caused by collision with a hard, blunt object, with resulting damage to the soft tissue. The rupture of capillaries and small blood vessels results in the seepage of blood under the skin, with pain, swelling and discoloration. Blows to the head, chest and abdomen should be watched carefully. Increased pulse rate, pallor and distressed breathing, as well as obvious deterioration, are signs that immediate allopathic intervention is needed.

The following remedies are useful in serious cases while allopathic attention is being sought

- Shock. Concussion with pallor, stupor or loss of consciousness.
  Arnica 6c, every 3–4 hours.
- Patient is blue and cold, and has a scanty sweat; does not want to be covered.
  Camphor 6c, every 3–4 hours.

- Patient is cold and blue with a profuse cold sweat.
  Veratrum album 6c, every 3–4 hours.
- The body is cold, face gray–yellow, the patient must have air.
  Carbo veg 6c, every 3–4 hours.

For different types of bruises

- To limit swelling and discoloration.
  Ice packs on the bruise, if applied immediately.
- On soft tissue when the skin is unbroken.
  Arnica tincture 1 in 10 on the skin.
  Arnica 6c internally, every 3–4 hours.
- On soft tissue when the skin is broken.
  Hamamelis tincture 1 in 10 on the skin.
  Hamamelis 6c internally, every 3–4 hours.

- On areas rich in nerves (e.g. base of neck or spine).
  Hypericum tincture 1 in 10 on the skin.
  Hypericum 6c, internally every 3–4 hours.
- Bruises to the breast.
  Bellis 6c, every 3–4 hours.

For bruises to eyes (black eyes)

- As a general treatment.
  Arnica tincture, diluted 1 in 10, on the bruise.
  Arnica 6c internally, every 3–4 hours.
- If arnica is not successful, or if the bruise is turning green.
  Ledum 6c, every 3–4 hours.

- For extreme pain in the eye itself.
  Hypericum 6c every 3–4 hours, or every time the pain returns.

For bruises to the bone surface

- As a general treatment.
  Symphytum 6c, every 3–4 hours.

- Jamming or crushing of fingers or toes.
  Hypericum 6c, every 3–4 hours.

Burns

It is customary to classify burns according to the damage that has been done. A **first degree** burn is only redness of the skin. **Second degree** burns involve blistering, while **third degree** burns involve damage to the deeper layers of the skin and the oozing of clear liquid from raw, inflamed areas. In **fourth degree** burns, destruction of the whole skin has occurred. Allopathic treatment should always be sought for burns of the third or fourth degree, and the patient should be kept covered and comfortable.

All burns are dangerous if not properly treated: the conditions to be aware of are infection, pain and shock. Clothing not adhering to severely burned areas should be cut away, but clothing burned into the flesh is most likely sterile and should not be removed.

TREATMENT

In severe burns, immediate applications of egg white, ice or honey are good emergency dressings. Cotton wool, oily substances and antiseptics are to be avoided. In less severe burns, a local dressing can be made with clean gauze. Saturate the gauze with Urtica tincture for first degree burns, and Hypericum tincture for second degree burns, 20 drops to a little water. Re-apply liquid often to keep dressing moist.

- Immediate treatment, first and second degree burns.
  Cold water or ice on the burn.
- Immediate treatment, third degree burns.
  Apply egg white liberally.
- When healing has started and pain subsided.
  *Apply a mixture of **Hypericum** and **Calendula** tinctures (**Hypercal**), diluted 1 in 10, locally.*
- For shock.
  Arnica 6c, every 1–2 hours.
- For persistent stinging.
  Urtica 30c, every time pain recurs.

- If there is fear of death, with anxiety and restlessness.
  Aconite 6c, every 30–60 minutes.
- For burns where the skin is red, shiny, hot and throbbing, and the pain is worsened by touching.
  Belladonna 6c, every 15–30 minutes.
- Burns when there is a swelling and sometimes looking like orange peel, with sensations of burning and stinging as if pricked by a hundred needles.
  Apis 6c, every 15–30 minutes.

- For second degree burns, with large blisters and intense pain.
  Cantharis 30c, every time pain recurs.
- Scarring third degree burns, with pains that are worse at night and soothed by warmth.
  Arsenicum alb 6c, every 3–4 hours.
- Deep burns of third degree, where yellow–green ulcers have formed.
  Kali bich 30c, every time pain recurs.
- For painful burns with a drawing, tightening sensation.
  Causticum 30c, every 3–4 hours.

Collapse

Collapse is always a serious incident, and should be regarded gravely. These remedies are included for emergency treatment only, while allopathic advice is being sought. Nevertheless they are very effective, and have produced many remarkable recoveries.

TREATMENT

- For shock immediately after an accident.
  Aconite 6c, every 30 minutes.
- For sudden and complete prostration, where the skin is dry and very cold, but the patient will not be covered or objects to it. Camphor is a good remedy for shock.
  Camphor 6c, every 30 minutes.
- For fainting or collapse, with cold sweat on the forehead and the whole body is icy cold.
  Veratrum album 6c, every 30 minutes.
- To reduce the prolonged effects of shock.
  Arnica 6c, every 3–4 hours.
- Patient is blue and cold; lies motionless as if dead, wants fresh air and to be fanned. Carbo veg is often called 'the corpse reviver' because of its success in collapse.
  Carbo veg 6c, every 30 minutes.
- For extreme weakness of the neck muscles, with heaviness of the head; the legs give out when walking, patient can hardly stand, walk or talk.
  Cocculus 6c, every 3–4 hours.
- Patient faints easily, from extremes of cold or heat, after getting wet, kneeling, and other minor causes.
  Sepia 6c, every 3–4 hours.

Concussion

Concussion is a special kind of bruising, where the brain has been bruised from a blow to the head. The symptoms vary, depending on the severity and extent of the injury. Mild cases may show no more than dizziness, passing off after an hour or two. In more serious cases the face and skin are pale, there are alterations in pulse rate and breathing, unequal pupil size and loss of consciousness. If vomiting occurs, ensure the airways are clear. There may be bleeding inside the mouth or throat. In very serious cases, symptoms are coma, diminished pulse and breathing, and cold extremities. In all cases of concussion other than mild ones allopathic advice should be sought.

TREATMENT

■ Loss of memory after concussion. *Arnica 200c* or *1M—from a practitioner.*

■ For concussion with resultant depression. *Nat sulph 200c—from a practitioner.*

■ Whether loss of consciousness has occurred or not. *Arnica 6c, every 30 minutes for 5 or 6 doses.*

Cuts and Scratches

Cuts and scratches are generally regarded as only skin deep, and require only antiseptic treatment. Deeper cuts may have divided not only the skin, but also structures underneath it such as ligaments and nerves, and in such cases surgical attention is necessary. Test to see if all normal movements can be carried out, and that there are no numb areas. Stitches will be needed if the wound is gaping and cannot be drawn together.

TREATMENT

First aid for cuts, scratches, and sharp wounds is substantially the same as for abrasions. Cleaning the wound is always necessary, but it is particularly important if it is an animal scratch. Suppuration (oozing of pus) should be watched cautiously, and allopathic advice should be sought if it worsens, and especially if the lymph nodes in the armpit, neck or groin become swollen or red streaks develop around the wound.

- For general purposes, externally.
  Hypercal (equal parts of calendula and hypericum tincture), applied undiluted locally or diluted 1 in 10.
- For clean-cut, deep or surgical cuts, with sharp stinging pain.
  Staphysagria 6c, every 3–4 hours.
- For inflammation locally.
  Hepar sulph 6c, every 3–4 hours.

- For sharp pain shooting up the limb.
  Hypericum 6c, every 3–4 hours.
- For wounds with suppuration, and where the patient has great sensitivity to the slightest touch.
  Hepar sulph 6c, every 3–4 hours.

Fracture

All fractures require allopathic treatment. Any suspected broken bones should be moved as little as possible, to prevent further injury. Fractures of the skull, neck or spine are usually the most dangerous. Bleeding from the ears, mouth, nose or into the eyes is often a sign of skull fracture. If the patient cannot move the fingers, the neck may be broken, while if they cannot move their legs, the back may be broken. In these cases, do not move the patient unless absolutely necessary, and call an ambulance. Fractures of arms or legs should be immobilised and allopathic treatment sought.

TREATMENT

- As a general treatment for trauma and bruising.
  Arnica 6c, every 3–4 hours.
- If nerve damage is involved, with shooting pains.
  Hypericum 6c, every 3–4 hours.
- As a general treatment, to aid knitting of the bones.
  Ruta grav 6c, every 3–4 hours.

- For aching, throbbing pain in bones.
  Eupatorium 6c, every 3–4 hours.
- For prickling pain as the bone is knitting.
  Symphytum 6c, every 3–4 hours.
- To promote the union of fractured bones.
  Calc phos 6x, a tissue salt, every 3–4 hours.

Puncture Wounds

This type of wound is usually caused by a nail, thorn, splinter or similarly sharp-pointed object. Although the wound may appear insignificant, deeper structures may be injured, or infection may be implanted. Damage to important organs, or large blood vessels, requires allopathic treatment.

Watch for tetanus. The typical case of tetanus occurs from a sharp but dirty object that punctures the skin and penetrates a short distance, with the wound closing over when the sharp object is withdrawn. The incubation period for tetanus (the time taken for any implanted tetanus infection to produce enough toxin to affect the spinal cord) may be anywhere from two to thirty days; the average is about ten. The longer the period of incubation, the milder the disease. After any untreated deep puncture wounds, tetanus should always be suspected if the patient complains of cramping, especially in the face or bowel. The following remedies can be used on puncture wounds while allopathic advice is being immediately sought.

TREATMENT

■ General treatment externally.
  Ledum tincture, 1 in 10 dilution.
■ General treatment internally.
  Ledum 6c, every 3–4 hours for a few days.

■ If the wound is painful, and there are shooting pains.
  Hypericum 6c, every 3–4 hours, or each time pain returns.

Sprains and Strains

Strains occur when the ligaments around a joint have been stretched, and sprains when they have been torn. The surrounding membranes of the joint may also be involved, resulting in fluid building up, which stretches the joint capsule and limits joint movement. In all cases, pain, swelling and discoloration occur. If the joint is badly displaced or wobbling, or impossible to straighten or bend, allopathic treatment is necessary, but can be followed with advantage by homoeopathic treatment.

Muscular problems, such as stiffness after unaccustomed exercise, have essentially the same treatment, so are covered here as well.

TREATMENT

- As a general treatment.
  *Apply **ice packs** immediately, externally.*
- For muscle strain after unaccustomed exercise, involving rupture, swelling and bruised pain.
  ***Arnica tincture**, diluted 1 in 10, applied locally as a firm compress; **Arnica 6c**, internally, every 3–4 hours.*

- For a sprain or strain of joint, with painful ligament, tendon or bone.
  ***Ruta grav tincture**, diluted 1 in 10, externally.*
  ***Ruta grav 6c**, internally, every 3–4 hours.*
- For painful muscle and tendons, from overexertion, with pain that is worse on initial motion and better on continued motion.
  ***Rhus tox 6c**, every 3–4 hours.*

Sunburn

Sunburn may lead to nothing more than a temporary reddening of the skin, or it may progress to blistering and deeper damage. It can be relieved temporarily by the application of aloe vera gel. Other external applications are as for burns; some internal remedies follow.

TREATMENT

- Sunburn with heat, redness and pain.
  ***Ferrum phos 6x**, a tissue salt, every 1–2 hours.*
- Sunburn with redness, heat and throbbing, worse from touch.
  ***Belladonna 6c**, every 1–2 hours until improved, then one dose every time the pain returns.*

- Sunburn, with large blisters, burning and containing clear or bloody liquid.
  ***Cantharis 30c**, every 3–4 hours for 1 day, then 1 dose every time the pain returns.*
- Sunburn peeling and leaving a raw, oozing surface, itching and burning.
  ***Bufo 6c**, every 1–2 hours.*

Sunstroke

Sunstroke, more correctly called **heatstroke**, is a disorder of the body's heat-regulating mechanism caused by overexposure to the sun or great heat, while in a humid atmosphere. It can also be brought about through excessive exercise. Sunstroke shows symptoms similar to heat exhaustion—both have headache, dizziness and weakness—but in sunstroke there is a high temperature and absence of sweating, while in heat exhaustion there is sweating with a normal or below normal temperature.

Sunstroke can be dangerous. The high temperature should be brought down as quickly as possible, as above 104°F (40°C) the person may collapse and become unconscious, with circulatory failure in severe cases. The immediate treatment is to bring down the temperature by wrapping the person in a wet sheet, and create a draught by fanning or switching on an electric fan. Keep the sheet wet and sponge the face. Once the person has cooled down, cover with a dry sheet: if the temperature begins to climb again, allopathic treatment is immediately necessary.

TREATMENT

General treatment should include giving a little water to drink, with half a teaspoon of salt added per half-litre of water, or an electrolyte replacer such as a sports drink. In stable cases, the following remedies can be used.

- Sunstroke with hot dizzy sensation and bursting pressure. Person anxious and restless, worse from sitting up. The skin is red and dry.
  Aconite 6c, every 30–60 minutes.
- Sunstroke with headache from the heat of the sun, with pounding head, flushed face and bloodshot eyes, person is bathed in sweat.
  Belladonna 6c, every 1–2 hours.
- Sunstroke with violent, pounding headache, pale face and fixed eyes, white tongue and laboured breathing.
  Glonoine 6c, every 2–3 hours.
- Hot, dry and inflamed, with flushed face and feverish symptoms.
  Ferrum phos 6x, a tissue salt, every 1–2 hours.
- Sunstroke with stupefied, giddy, intoxicated feeling and band-like pain around the head.
  Gelsemium 6c, every 2–3 hours.

■ Collapse after overexposure to the sun, with great coldness. *Camphor 6c*, *every 30 minutes.*

■ Headache after sun exposure, like a thousand tiny hammers, with debility and thirst. *Nat mur 6x*, *a tissue salt, every 1–2 hours.*

4
Common Problems

Acne

Acne is a common problem in adolescents but also often occurs in adults. It is thought to be due to hormonal imbalances, and perhaps faulty diet. It appears as inflamed oil glands, generally on the skin of the face, neck or back, which have become blocked and often infected. The pimples are raised, red and usually pus-filled; blackheads are common. The pimples may or may not be painful.

TREATMENT

External treatment of the skin should be as gentle as possible, avoiding harsh antiseptic soaps. Creams and ointments containing antibiotics or the cortisone type of hormones should not be used, since general allergic reactions and permanent damage to the skin can easily occur.

Avoid chocolate, cheese, nuts, soft drinks and junk food. Supplementation with vitamins A and B[6], and the mineral zinc, is beneficial. The most suitable remedy given below should be tried for three to six weeks.

■ Painful pimples with a small area of white pus in the centre. *Eugenia jambosa 6c, every 3–4 hours.*

■ Pustular acne, only on the cheeks and nose. *Ledum 6c, every 3–4 hours.*

- Oily skin with small pimples and blackheads in adolescents, following mental strain or sexual frustration.
  Selenium 6c, every 3–4 hours.
- Pimples on the forehead and other areas where the skin is thin.
  Calc pic 6c, every 3–4 hours.
- Blind boils and burning stinging acne, mainly on the face, chest and shoulders, in restless, depressed and worried adolescents.
  Kali brom 6c, every 3–4 hours.
- Lesions contain pus, are of a purplish hue, are hard, painful and often symmetrical.
  Arnica 6c, every 3–4 hours.
- Pimples that leave a raised scar after healing.
  Graphites 6c, every 3–4 hours.
- Large numbers of pimples that heal leaving purple–red scars and pits.
  Ant tart 6c, every 3–4 hours.
- Weeping pustules, forming yellow crusts, that will not heal.
  Calc sulph 6x, a tissue salt, every 3–4 hours.
- Painful red pustules like small boils, highly sensitive, discharging yellow pus.
  Hepar sulph 6c, every 3–4 hours.
- Pimples that come to a head but will not discharge, or discharge leaving a scar.
  Silicea 6x, a tissue salt, every 3–4 hours.
- Long-standing acne, with rough hard skin, made worse by washing and heat.
  Sulphur 6c, every 3–4 hours.

Acne Rosacea

Acne rosacea is the name for acne-like symptoms that occur in middle age, with red, thickened skin, blotchy red patches due to the enlargement of small blood vessels and appearing as red, pus-filled spots. There is easy flushing of the nose and cheeks, at first periodically, then permanently. Possible causes are thought to be oral contraceptives, steroid ointments, and possibly a deficiency of vitamin B[2].

TREATMENT

- As a general treatment.
  Avoid hot spicy foods, tea, coffee and alcohol. Reduce stress as much as possible. Supplement with B complex vitamins.
- When the face is always red and dry, with pimples and pus-filled spots.
  Sulphur iod 6c, every 3–4 hours.

- In the early stages, when the face is red, dry, and burning hot.
  Belladonna 6c, every 3–4 hours.
- There is burning and stinging of the lesions, often in women with flushing or scanty periods, and the condition is always worse in heat.
  Sanguinaria 6c, every 3–4 hours.
- The face is dry and burning, and condition is worse from cold applications; there is flaky, scaly skin.
  Arsenicum alb 6c, every 3–4 hours.
- When the acne has a symmetrical look on cheeks and forehead.
  Arnica 6c, every 3–4 hours.
- For red, painful or itchy spots, where the face is puffy and swollen and the acne is worse in cold or wet weather.
  Rhus tox 6c, every 3–4 hours.
- Where the face is reddish–purple and mottled, patient feels worse in the morning, after sleep or from exposure to the sun.
  Lachesis 12c, morning and evening.
- In older people, with poor circulation, distended veins, and blue extremities. The acne gives no sensation of heat.
  Carbo animalis 6c, every 3–4 hours.

Anemia

Anemia is a deficiency in the blood, either in quality or quantity. It is usually a decrease in the number of red blood cells, or a reduction in their hemoglobin content. Symptoms include pale face, fingernail beds and mucous membranes, general fatigue and weakness, and shortness of breath. There are several possible causes, but the most significant are excessive loss of blood, such as may be caused by very heavy menstrual bleeding, childbirth, gastrointestinal disease or an accident, and inadequate intake of iron. Vitamin B^{12} is the missing factor in pernicious anemia.

TREATMENT

The first action is to supplement the diet with extra iron, either through iron-rich foods such as red meat and parsley, or by iron supplements. Often, however, there can be problems with the absorption and assimilation of this iron into the red blood cells; in such cases the following remedies can be of great use.

- In simple anemia, to help with assimilation of dietary iron.
  Ferrum phos 6x, a tissue salt, every 3–4 hours.
- Anmia due to blood loss, with chilliness, digestive distress and exhaustion.
  China 6c, every 3–4 hours.
- Anemia with depression of spirits and prostration, headache, constipation, dry mouth and lips, and tendency to cold sores.
  Nat mur 6x, a tissue salt, every 3–4 hours.
- Patient is robust-looking, but the face is pale, flushing easily.
  Ferrum met 6c, every 3–4 hours.
- In children and adolescents, during growth spurts, or during convalescence.
  Calc phos 6x, a tissue salt, every 3–4 hours.
- Anemia coupled with mental overload.
  Picric acid 6c, every 3–4 hours.

Anxiety

Sudden, short-lived anxiety due to particular circumstances is natural and needs no treatment, since after a short time the mind and body return to normal. Apprehension and worry that continue longer with less cause, coupled with increased pulse rate, clammy skin and disturbed sleep and appetite, warrant attention. Treatment with tranquilizers has short-term value, and over the longer term carries the risk of side effects and dependence. Those taking tranquilizers and who wish to take homeopathic medicines should wean themselves off their medication very gently, as extreme reactions can occur if tranquilizers are stopped suddenly.

TREATMENT

- Anxious after nervous stress, patient cannot relax or sleep easily, is irritable and jumps at the slightest sound.
  Kali phos 6x, a tissue salt, every 3–4 hours.
- Patient is oversensitive to many influences, with anxiety, repeated sighing, insomnia, palpitations and loss of appetite; he or she is better when the mind is occupied. Often the after effect of an emotional shock.
  Ignatia 6c, every 3–4 hours.

- Anxiety, with restlessness and fear of death, often at the onset of an acute illness.
  Aconite 6c, every 3–4 hours.
- Anxiety before any ordeal, such as performing in front of an audience, in tense intellectual types who are irritable and touchy, lacking confidence and intolerant of contradiction.
  Lycopodium 6c, every 3–4 hours.
- Anxiety with restlessness, exhaustion and desire for warmth, patient fends off anxiety by being meticulously tidy.
  Arsenicum album 6c, every 3–4 hours.
- Nervous, agitated and restless; sufferer walks faster from anxiety. Hurried and anxious before appointments, torments from anticipation of failure.
  Argentum nit 6c, every 3–4 hours.

- Extremely sensitive to atmospheres, thunderstorms, the thoughts and feelings of others, and to touch. Nervous and fidgety, desires affection and gives it easily.
  Phosphorus 6c, every 3–4 hours.
- Patient is easily anxious and discouraged, apprehensive and fearful; feels very chilly, yet sweats easily about the head and feet.
  Calc carb 6c, every 3–4 hours.
- Nervous, irritable and stubborn person, yet thin and weak and exhausted easily by effort; has anxiety before events; fears failure.
  Silicea 6x, a tissue salt, every 3–4 hours.

Appetite Problems

Problems with appetite are often ephemeral, and are usually related to other symptoms of the time. Nevertheless, a few remedies have well-defined symptom pictures, and are often useful.

TREATMENT

- Appetite varies: from good to complete loss.
  Ferrum phos 6x, a tissue salt, every 3–4 hours.

- Appetite excessive, even at night, but easily satisfied.
  Lycopodium 6c, every 3–4 hours.

- Appetite variable, from voracious to indifferent. Child wants things, but rejects when offered, with irritability. Grinds teeth at night. *Cina 6c, every 3–4 hours.*

- Appetite absent, with irritability, especially after excesses of living. *Nux vomica 6c, every 3–4 hours.*

Arthritis

Arthritis is a disorder affecting the structure of the joints and their surrounding tissue. There is pain, swelling and, frequently, changes in the joint structure. The condition usually begins in the small joints of the hands, especially the fingers, although other joints can be involved. With recurrent attacks, the joints can become swollen and immobile. There can often be wasting of the surrounding muscle. General treatments of benefit include compresses on the affected parts and an alkaline diet.

The term arthritis covers more than a hundred different types of joint disease, the most common being rheumatoid arthritis and osteoarthritis. Rheumatoid arthritis is an inflammatory disease where the joint tissues are attacked by the body's own defenses. It is most often seen as a shifting attack on one or more joints at a time, frequently settling on the fingers, but sometimes involving many joints in increasing pain, swelling and immobility.

Osteoarthritis is a degeneration of the joints that is most likely to strike those that receive the most use or stress over the years. As a result, the knees, big toes, spine, and end joints of the fingers are common sites of complaint. Symptoms vary from mild to severe depending on the amount of degeneration that has taken place. It is caused by the disintegration of the cartilage that covers the ends of the bone, which leaves roughened surfaces and results in stiffness and pain.

TREATMENT

- In acute attacks, when the joint is swollen, painful and red, aggravated by motion. *Ferrum phos 6x, a tissue salt, every 3–4 hours.*

- Pain with sour-smelling sweat and a persistent creamy coating on the back of the tongue. *Nat phos 6x, a tissue salt, every 3–4 hours.*

- Pain and stiffness, often brought on by cold and damp and improved by heat. Pains are worse on initial movement, especially in the morning, but better after limbering up.
Rhus tox 6c, every 3–4 hours.
- For a stabbing pain that is better when absolutely still, worse on movement and in dry, cold weather, and is relieved by pressure being applied and lying on the affected part.
Bryonia 6c, every 3–4 hours.
- Joint pain made worse by heat and warm rooms, flitting from one part of the body to another.
Pulsatilla 6c, every 3–4 hours.
- Joints feel cold and numb, with pain and stiffness increasing when the weather changes.
Calc phos 6x, a tissue salt, every 3–4 hours.
- Pain mainly in the jaw and neck, with muscle spasm, better in warm, damp or humid weather.
Causticum 6c, every 3–4 hours.
- Aches and pains that are worse at night; there is greasy, offensive sweat and a foul taste in the mouth in the morning.
Mercurius 6c, every 3–4 hours.

- Pain and stiffness that is worse in cold, damp weather, especially after becoming overheated.
Dulcamara 6c, every 3–4 hours.
- Stiff, bruised pains after injury, no matter how long ago.
Arnica 6c, every 3–4 hours.
- Bruised, sore, aching stiffness, sufferer feels they must move, but feels no better when they do.
Phytolacca 6c, every 3–4 hours.
- Pain is worse when at rest and improved by movement, and is particularly aggravated by the approach of stormy weather.
Rhododendron 6c, every 3–4 hours.
- Limbs are stiff and painful after becoming cold, or when the weather changes from warm to cold; condition is somewhat improved by moving about.
Dulcamara 6c, every 3–4 hours.
- Pain with great creaking of the joints.
Nat mur 6x, a tissue salt, every 3–4 hours.
- Pain in the joints, especially the larger ones, where the tendons meet the bone, condition is improved by warmth.
Ruta grav 6c, every 3–4 hours.

Asthma

The symptoms of asthma are attacks of breathlessness, brought about by contraction of the bronchial tubes, with the secretion of a very thick, sticky mucus instead of normal fluid phlegm. Attacks vary greatly in frequency, duration and intensity, ranging from occasional periods of wheezing and breathing difficulty, to severe attacks that almost cause suffocation. Most of the symptoms arise from an allergic or hypersensitivity reaction taking place in the bronchial walls.

TREATMENT

A great improvement can often be seen by following a diet free of dairy products, wheat, oats, rye and barley. Other allergens, such as dusts and pollens, can also cause asthma, and can be treated by homeopathic desensitisation. The following remedies are also of great use: they should be taken often during an attack, and 2–3 times a day between attacks. Serious attacks always need allopathic attention.

■ Attack comes on suddenly after midnight, with anxiety, restlessness and thirst, often after exposure to dry cold wind.
Aconite 6c, *every 1–2 hours.*

■ Constriction of the chest, with spasms of the bronchial muscles, and spasmodic dry tickling cough. Difficulty breathing when lying down.
Mag phos 6x, *a tissue salt, every 1–2 hours.*

■ Asthma in children, who wake with cough, profuse sweating, mouth breathing, and sensation of intense suffocation.
Sambucus 6c, *every 30–60 minutes.*

■ Asthma worsened from exposure to house dust and dust mite.
Blatta 6c, *every 3–4 hours.*

■ Nervous asthma, and from taking the least food, with depressed nervous system. Attacks with oppressed breathing.
Kali phos 6x, *a tissue salt, every 1–2 hours.*

■ Asthma with gagging: may have persistent nausea and vomiting, but feel no better by it.
Ipecac 6c, *every 1–2 hours.*

■ Asthma with muscle spasms in chest and arms, perhaps vomiting after each spasm.
Cuprum met 6c, *every 1–2 hours.*

■ Asthma with white-coated tongue and coughing up white mucus with difficulty.
Kali mur 6x, *a tissue salt, every 1–2 hours.*

- Asthma with expectoration of clear, frothy mucus and watery discharges from the eyes and nose.
  Nat mur 6x, a tissue salt, every 1–2 hours.
- Attacks between midnight and 3 a.m., with burning in the chest, restlessness, and anxiety, sufferer wants sips of water, is better by sitting up.
  Arsenicum 6c, every 1–2 hours.
- Asthma worse around 3 a.m., with exhaustion, pale face, and great rattling of mucus in chest, hard to raise.
  Ant tart 6c, every 1–2 hours.
- Asthma is worse 2–4 a.m., with chilliness; may have stabbing pains. Sufferer sits bending forward, or with arms on knees.
  Kali carb 6c, every 1–2 hours.
- Asthma worse from going to bed, or shortly after going to sleep.
  Aralia racemosa 6c, every 3–4 hours.
- Whistling asthma towards 3 a.m., with irritating cough and severe congestion, difficult to expectorate.
  Ammonium carb 6c, every 1–2 hours.
- Asthma worse 3–5 a.m., in damp conditions, with early morning diarrhoea.
  Nat sulph 6x, a tissue salt, every 3–4 hours.
- Asthma in obese, cold-sensitive persons, worse 3–5 a.m. and from humidity.
  Thuja 6c, every 3–4 hours.
- Asthma worse on waking in the morning, with great fear of constriction.
  Lachesis 12c, morning and evening.

$\mathcal{B}ad \; \mathcal{B}reath$

Bad breath can have many causes, including decayed teeth, sinus problems, tonsillitis, bronchitis, indigestion, constipation, liver trouble, and strong smelling ingredients in the diet such as garlic. It usually occurs as part of a broader symptom picture, but a few remedies are helpful.

TREATMENT

- Bad breath especially in morning, with thirst.
  Mercurius 6c, every 3–4 hours.
- Bad breath with irritability in the mornings, especially after overeating or alcohol.
  Nux vomica 6c, every 3–4 hours.

Biliousness

Biliousness is a rather vague term applied sometimes to indigestion with irrritability, vague nausea, headache and constipation. It may occur after overindulgence in rich food or drink, and often after excessive production of bile from the liver.

TREATMENT

■ Biliousness with greenish–brown coated tongue, sallow skin, and a yellow tinge to the eyes. There may be a bitter taste, and vomiting of bile or bitter fluid. *Nat sulph 6x, a tissue salt, every 3–4 hours.*

■ Biliousness after over-indulgence in food or drink, with irritability, worse in the morning. Seeks coffee and stimulants. *Nux vomica 6c, every 3–4 hours.*

■ Biliousness with a white-coated tongue or light-colored stools. *Kali mur 6x, a tissue salt, every 3–4 hours.*

■ Biliousness with nausea, inclination to vomit, wants hot water or hot drinks. Yellow tinge to the skin, and pain under the right shoulder blade. *Chelidonium 6c, every 3–4 hours.*

Boils and Abscesses

An abscess is formed when the body reacts to an infection with redness, heat, swelling, pain and tenderness, and often an accumulation of pus. Abscesses can occur anywhere: they are usually very painful and should not be squeezed. On the surface of the skin, an abscess also forms the familiar congested area called a **boil**; it may also develop from a spreading ulcer. If the infected area has several openings or heads, a **carbuncle** is forming, and allopathic advice should be sought. Any area showing uncontrollable suppuration should also receive allopathic treatment.

- Immediate treatment.
  Apply **Hypercal** *externally, diluted 1 in 10.*
  Internally give **Calendula 6c,** *every 3–4 hours.*
- In the early stages of inflammation, when there is heat, pain, congestion and fever.
  Ferrum phos 6x, *a tissue salt, every 3–4 hours.*
- For the swelling, before pus has begun to form.
  Kali mur 6x, *a tissue salt, every 3–4 hours.*
- Skin hot, red, painful and throbbing, with general restlessness.
  Belladonna 6c *every 3–4 hours.*
- Skin shining and swollen, with stinging pains that are worse from heat.
  Apis 6c, *every 3–4 hours.*
- Boils intolerably painful and sensitive. Patient is chilly, but boil is hot.
  Hepar sulph 6c, *every 3–4 hours.*
- Purplish wounds, burning and throbbing. To hasten resolution.
  Tarentula 12c, *once a day.*
- Boils slow in coming to a head, to hasten resolution.
  Hepar sulph 6c, *every 3–4 hours, or* **Silicea 6x,** *a tissue salt, every 3–4 hours.*
- When suppuration and discharge have occurred, but are slow to clear.
  Silicea 6x, *a tissue salt, every 3–4 hours.*
- If the discharge occurs too long, and the wound refuses to heal.
  Calc sulph 6x, *a tissue salt, every 3–4 hours.*
- Unhealthy skin, easily infected and sensitive to touch.
  Hepar sulph 6c, *every 3–4 hours.*
- When even minor wounds turn septic, and develop into boils.
  Silicea 6x, *a tissue salt, every 3–4 hours.*

Bone Pain

Bone pain can show a variety of types and have a variety of causes, from the sharp pain of fracture, to the aching pain of influenza and the dull pain of arthritis. Occasionally bone pain can also be due to a dietary deficiency. Any pain that fails to clear should receive professional assessment.

- Prickling pains in the bone, especially after a fracture, when the bone is knitting.
  Symphytum 6c, every 3–4 hours.
- Bones ache, are numb, chilly; feel great weakness when climbing stairs.
  Calc phos 6x, a tissue salt, every 3–4 hours.
- Bruised, throbbing pain in the bones and especially in the eye sockets, during fever or flu.
  Eupatorium 6c, every 3–4 hours.
- Bone pain worse from any movement, better by lying completely still.
  Bryonia 6c, every 3–4 hours.

- Pain on the surface of bones, often with spurs or bony outgrowths such as bunions.
  Calc fluor 6x, a tissue salt, every 3–4 hours.
- To promote the union of fractured bones, to shorten the duration of the pain.
  Calc phos 6x, every 3–4 hours.
- Bone pain with easy sweating, especially around the feet. Ulceration of bone.
  Silicea 6x, a tissue salt, every 3–4 hours.

$\mathscr{B}$ronchitis

Bronchitis is an inflammation of the mucous membranes of the bronchial tubes. It often follows a cold or influenza, and may become chronic. The usual symptoms are fever with a harsh, dry cough, chest pain and wheezing, although the chest pain improves when expectoration begins. If the temperature rises above 102°F (39°C), or breathing becomes rapid and difficult, or the phlegm contains blood, allopathic treatment is essential.

TREATMENT

- Heat and congestion, with short painful cough and oppressed breathing. Discharge is absent or clear and minimal, may show traces of blood.
  Ferrum phos 6x, a tissue salt, every 3–4 hours.

- Bronchitis that may come on suddenly, with fever, restlessness and anxiety. Dry staccato cough, with notable thirst.
  Aconite 6c, every 1–2 hours.

- Sudden onset, with high fever, restlessness, pounding headache and flushed face. Cough is worse at night and when lying down. *Belladonna 6c, every 1–2 hours.*
- Expectoration is thick, yellow and heavy. The cough is made better by heat and warm drinks, but aggravated by cold drinks. *Silicea 6x, a tissue salt, every 3–4 hours.*
- Dry, stabbing painful cough, with chest pain relieved by holding tightly or lying on it. *Bryonia 6c, every 3–4 hours.*
- Expectoration is thick, white, tenacious and the tongue has a white or grayish-white coating. *Kali mur 6x, a tissue salt, every 3–4 hours.*
- Loose and rattling cough, patient is sensitive to drafts, worse in the evening and on lying down, better from warm and humid air. *Hepar sulph 6c, every 3–4 hours.*
- Tight, ticklish cough, with traces of blood. Burning in the chest, with craving for cold water. *Phosphorus 6c, every 3–4 hours.*
- Phlegm is light yellow, watery and copious, or greenish and slimy, with back of the tongue coated yellow. There is a craving for fresh air. *Kali sulph 6x, a tissue salt, every 3–4 hours.*
- Bronchitis with loose and rattling expectoration of clear, watery mucus. *Nat mur 6x, a tissue salt, every 3–4 hours.*
- Thick, bland, creamy expectoration, loose in the mornings but dry at night. *Pulsatilla 6c, every 3–4 hours.*
- Expectoration of thick, clear, jelly-like mucus, especially in anemic persons. *Calc phos 6x, a tissue salt, every 3–4 hours.*

Catarrh

Catarrh is the excessive discharge of mucus from any mucous membrane, but most commonly the nose, sinuses and lungs. It is the attempt by the body to protect itself against invasion by pathogens, as a reaction against irritation, and to rid itself of toxic wastes that are not being properly eliminated by the kidneys, bowel or skin. Homeopathy regards chronic catarrh as a symptom of general body toxicity, which should be treated by deeper acting, more constitutional remedies. The following remedies are for more acute conditions, and can be used primarily according to the colour of the mucus discharge.

TREATMENT

- First stage, with fever, inflammation, heat and a clear or minimal discharge, occasionally tinged with blood.
  Ferrum phos 6x, *a tissue salt, every 3–4 hours.*

- Catarrh with a watery, frothy, clear discharge, often with sneezing. There may be great thirst, or complete absence of it, and a loss of smell and taste.
  Nat mur 6x, *a tissue salt, every 3–4 hours.*

- Second stage of catarrhal discharge, with thick white mucus that is bland and abundant. Tongue is coated white.
  Kali mur 6x, *a tissue salt, every 3–4 hours.*

- Yellow or white discharge that is thick, stringy and ropy, or with tough and jelly-like plugs, with feeling of pressure around the bridge of the nose.
  Kali bich 6c, *every 3–4 hours.*

- Bronchial catarrh, with coughing up tiny, yellow, tough lumps of mucus.
  Calc fluor 6x, *a tissue salt, every 3–4 hours.*

- Profuse thick, yellow discharge, the inside of the nose is sore and ulcerated; sneezing makes symptoms worse.
  Arsenicum iod 6c, *every 3–4 hours.*

- Third stage of discharge, with yellow mucus that is watery or slimy. Tongue is yellow at the back; person feels better in the fresh air.
  Kali sulph 6x, *a tissue salt, every 3–4 hours.*

- Yellowish discharge, with sore scabs and fissures inside the nose, made worse by blowing. Sense of smell is abnormally acute.
  Graphites 6c, *every 3–4 hours.*

- Bright yellow discharge, running all the time, with mucus dripping down the back of the throat, and small ulcers in the nose.
  Hydrastis 6c, *every 3–4 hours.*

- Bland mucus, yellow or greenish–yellow, that is changeable in colour and stops and starts, with loss of smell and taste. Patient is worse in stuffy rooms and better outdoors.
  Pulsatilla 6c, *every 3–4 hours.*

- Mucus is thick, yellow or greenish–yellow, often offensive, and sometimes mixed with blood. *Cal sulph 6x, a tissue salt, every 3–4 hours.*
- Thick offensive discharge, yellow and slimy, sometimes streaked with blood. Skin has a greasy sweat. *Merc sol 6c, every 3–4 hours.*
- Profuse secretion of greenish mucus with tongue green–gray at the back. Worse in the damp and at every change of weather. *Nat sulph 6x, a tissue salt, every 3–4 hours.*

- Dry scabs inside the nose that bleed easily, nose stuffier indoors than out of doors, cold sores on the outside of the nose. *Sulphur 6c, every 3–4 hours.*
- Chronic catarrh, with offensive discharge, excessive sweating of the feet, and poor resistance to infection. The edge of the nostrils is dry and ulcerated. The tip of nose may itch. *Silicea 6x, a tissue salt, every 3–4 hours.*

Chilblains and Poor Circulation

Poor circulation includes persistently cold hands and feet, and cold, mottled skin. Chilblains are a special case of poor circulation, where the cold has caused a constriction of the blood vessels in areas such as the fingers, toes, ears and nose; here the tissue becomes purple or deep red, begins to itch and burn, and is painful. Exercise and massage help to improve the circulation.

TREATMENT

General treatments for poor circulation
- Poor circulation, with intense chilliness, always worse from drafts. *Hepar sulph 6c, every 3–4 hours.*

- Poor circulation, patient faints easily, with chilliness, especially in the evening. *Sepia 6c, every 3–4 hours.*

Remedies for chilblains

- As an external application. *Tincture of Tamus can be applied locally, morning and evening.*
- Chilblains, to prevent appearance. *Calc phos 6x, a tissue salt, every 3–4 hours daily during autumn and winter.*
- Chilblains that are hot, red, congested and throbbing. *Belladonna 6c, every 3–4 hours.*
- Chilblains itchy, swollen, with stinging pain. *Apis 6c, every 3–4 hours.*

- Chilblains itching, burning bluish–red and swollen; become worse from warmth and in bed. *Pulsatilla 6c, every 3–4 hours.*
- Chilblains, with sore, swollen and bruised pain. *Arnica 6c, every 3–4 hours.*
- Broken chilblains exuding thin, yellow fluid. *Kali sulph 6x, a tissue salt, every 3–4 hours.*

Cold Sores

Cold sores are an infection of the herpes simplex virus, showing usually as itching, burning blisters inside the mouth and on the lips, chin or cheeks. When ruptured the blisters leave a thin, yellowish crust, often with broken skin or fissures, that is very prone to secondary infection. While the symptoms may clear up after 5–10 days, the virus is not destroyed, but incubates until conditions are ripe for recurrence. Triggering factors for recurrence include stress, emotional trauma and any general lowering of resistance.

TREATMENT

Lysine (an amino acid) can be taken as a supplement, along with zinc and bioflavonoids. Avoid grains, seeds, peanuts and chocolate.

Externally, apply ice as often as possible in the very early stages. Applications of tea tree oil are also useful for aborting attacks. After the lesions have formed, solanum nigrum ointment is soothing.

- As a general preventative, if infection or recurrence is suspected. *Herpes simplex nosode 30c, morning and evening for a few days.*

- Large blisters that smart and burn intensely, may also bleed. *Cantharis 6c, every 3–4 hours.*

- Deep crack in middle of lower lip, mouth very dry, pearl-like blisters on the lips.
  Nat mur 6x, a tissue salt, every 3–4 hours.
- Corners of the mouth ulcerate; angry-looking blisters with great itching and tingling.
  Rhus tox 6c, every 3–4 hours.
- Many ulcers inside the mouth, very sore and worse at night, with easily bleeding gums.
  Sempervivum 6c, every 3–4 hours.
- Cracks at the corners of the mouth, lips pale, red itchy rash on chin, burning blisters on tongue, breath foul.
  Capsicum 6c, every 3–4 hours.

Colds

The common cold is known medically as **coryza,** an inflammation of the nasal mucosa, and is considered by allopaths to be due to a virus. The symptom picture normally goes through a number of stages as the disorder progresses. Its symptoms are sneezing, discharge from the nose and eyes, and often sore and reddened eyes. It differs from **influenza** in that there is no bone pain, less prostration, and less sweat. In homeopathic treatment the color and effect of the discharges are important, as well as the influences that make the disorder better or worse.

Stages
1 Mucous membrane inflammation and pain. Discharge is absent or minimal.
2 Running of the nose, clear and more profuse, changing to white as the disorder progresses. Eye involvement. Sneezing.
3 Discharge thickening in texture, and moving from white to yellow.
4 Discharge yellow to yellow–green.

TREATMENT

The homeopathic treatment of colds is very effective, and can stop a cold at any stage. Since colds can have differing symptom pictures, careful prescribing is necessary. As general winter treatment, daily doses of half a gram of vitamin C to children aged 7–14, and one gram to anyone over fourteen, is useful in preventing infection and hastening recovery.

- To build up the general health after a cold.

Stage 1 colds

Mucous membrane inflammation and pain. Discharge is absent or minimal.

- In the very early stages, where there is the sensation of icy cold, but no fever. Nose stopped, dry and contracted. The head aches in front.
  Camphor 6c, every 2 hours for a few doses is enough.
- After exposure to dry cold; not much running of the nose, but burning and pricking of the throat, restlessness and heat, obvious fever. Anxiety, apprehension and fear.
  Aconite 6c, even every 20 minutes.
- High temperature with sudden onset, dry mucous membranes and great congestion of the nose and throat. Profuse sweating, restlessness, flushed face.
  Belladonna 6c, every 3–4 hours.
- For a cold beginning with sneezing.
  Nat mur 6x, a tissue salt, every 3–4 hours.

- *Calc phos 6x, a tissue salt, every 3–4 hours.*
- Painful, dry or moist cough. May be sneezing, but no other discharges. Feverishness; face pale or flushed, pulse is rapid.
  Ferrum phos 6x, a tissue salt, every 3–4 hours.
- The nose remains dry and obstructed, headache over the root of the nose persists, and is aggravated by motion. The lips are dry and there is considerable thirst for water in large amounts, but not particularly often.
  Bryonia 6c, every 3–4 hours.
- The nose is dry and blocked at night, flowing in the morning and in a warm room, with a sore throat. Shivering if uncovered, can't get warm enough, wants warm drinks, very irritable.
  Nux vomica 6c, every 3–4 hours.

Stage 2 colds

Running of the nose, clear and more profuse, changing to white as the disorder progresses. Eye involvement. Sneezing. Hay fever symptoms.

- Clear, profuse and acrid discharge from the nose, corroding the nostrils and upper lip, with heat and burning. Eyes are suffused and watery, tears are bland. There is sneezing and headache.
  Allium cepa 6c, every 3–4 hours.
- Tears are burning and acrid, the nasal discharge bland. Conjunctivitis, worse from light; the patient often dabs at the eyes repeatedly. The coryza is worse at night, in a warm room, and from lying down; better in the fresh air.
  Euphrasia 6c, every 3–4 hours.

- Thin, watery, nasal discharge irritating the upper lip, but better in a warm room. The discharge is more burning in character; the throat also burns. The patient may feel intensely hot, yet craves heat—hot drinks, hot rooms, hot applications—and is restless, always worse around midnight. *Arsenicum 6c, every 3–4 hours.*
- White mucus discharge, with stuffiness and congestion. *Kali mur 6x, a tissue salt, every 3–4 hours.*

- Often good for treating a cold that begins by sneezing. Abundant tears and nasal discharge, clear and watery or thick and white—like the white of an egg, either raw or cooked, sneezing is violent, paroxysmal, loss of smell and taste, dry cracked lips, cold sores about lips and nose. *Nat mur 6x, a tissue salt, every 3–4 hours.*

Stage 3 colds

Discharge thickening in texture, and moving from white to yellow.

- Bland, thick yellow discharges, often at the end of a head cold. The nose is stopped up indoors and at night, discharging in the open air. There is often a loss of smell and taste. The lips are chapped and peel easily; patient has a dry mouth with no thirst and a generally poor appetite. Better in open air, and worse from heat. *Pulsatilla 6c, every 3–4 hours.*
- Violent coryza, with red swollen throat, hoarse, raw and rough voice, better after beginning to talk. Thick yellow, offensive mucus, sneezing and coughing. Thirst for cold drinks, especially at night, but generally better from heat. *Rhus tox 6c, every 3–4 hours.*

- For colds that invariably spread to the throat, or where every sore throat ends in a cold. There is constant, profuse salivation with intense thirst, bad breath and bad taste in the mouth. The nasal discharge is thin, with sneezing, watering of the eyes and a sore throat that stings and pricks, making swallowing difficult. The nostrils can be red, raw and ulcerated. Often there is a profuse, offensive sweat, which does not relieve the symptoms. *Mercurius 6c, every 3–4 hours.*
- Discharge is yellow, patient has desire for fresh air. *Kali sulph 6x, a tissue salt, every 3–4 hours.*

Stage 4 colds

Discharge yellow to yellow–green.

■ Takes cold at slightest exposure to fresh air, generally unhealthy. Nose blocks on going outside, with a thin, irritating discharge, yellow to yellow–green in color. A sore throat usually accompanies the discharge, is very sensitive to touch and drafts, often with the sensation of a splinter there. Sometimes a loose and barking cough, usually worse at night. Cold sores are common.
Hepar sulph 6c, every 3–4 hours.

■ Yellow discharges changing to yellow–green, profuse and intermittent, slimy and tenacious, sometimes tinged with blood.
Calc sulph 6x, a tissue salt, every 3–4 hours.

■ Catarrh, with thick yellow (or green), stringy, ropy discharge, or tough and jelly-like; can be drawn into long strings.
Kali bich 6c, every 3–4 hours.

■ Stringy, yellow, nasal discharge, sticky and tenacious.
Hydrastis 6c, every 3–4 hours.

Colitis

Colitis is inflammation of the colon. It may show as four different conditions, which have some symptoms in common. There are varying degrees of abdominal pain, constipation, diarrhea and bloating after meals. If blood appears in the stool professional advice should be sought.

■ **Irritable colon** involves overactivity of an otherwise normal bowel, with bouts of diarrhea and an increased frequency of bowel movements, with or without pain. These bouts are usually related to stressful emotions, overtiredness and mental and physical stress.

■ **Spastic colon** shows as very painful spasms of the colon, which are brought on by foods or laxatives, and which may be relieved by passing wind or stool.

■ **Mucous colitis** is a condition where the bowel movements are covered by clear mucus, or joined together by mucus strands, or where large lumps of clear mucus can be passed alone.

■ **Ulcerative colitis** is a potentially dangerous condition, where the colon becomes ulcerated. It may involve fever, pain, profuse bloody diarrhea and varying amounts of mucus in the stool. There may be marked loss of weight and general debility.

TREATMENT

- Loose bowel movments every morning, with spasms of pain, often after nervous stress or emotional trauma.
  Ignatia 6c, every 3–4 hours.
- Painless diarrhea, with distension of the whole abdomen, which is tender and rumbling.
  China 6c, every 3–4 hours.
- Stools liquid but containing hard lumps, with belching of undigested food and white-coated tongue.
  Ant crud 6c, every 3–4 hours.
- Abdominal pain with offensive gas. Passing of dry, bulky stool covered in mucus, or joined together by strings of mucus.
  Graphites 6c, every 3–4 hours.

- Sudden cramping pain, worse after eating and improved by bending double or applying heat and pressure to the abdomen.
  Colocynthis 6c, every 3–4 hours.
- Burning pains in abdomen with vomiting and diarrhea. Desire for warmth and warm drinks. Often worse midnight to 3 a.m.
  Arsenicum album 6c, every 3–4 hours.
- Cutting abdominal pain, not relieved by passing stool, with hot offensive stools accompanied by blood and mucus.
  Mercurius 6c, every 3–4 hours.
- Diarrhea with blood, gushing like a fire hydrant; anus feels wide open afterwards.
  Phosphorus 6c, every 3–4 hours.

Conjunctivitis

Conjunctivitis is the inflammation of the tissue lining the eyelid and eye, due usually to cold, irritation or infection. It is often accompanied by redness of the eyeball, gushes of tears or a yellow discharge, particularly noticeable in the mornings. The eyes may be cleaned using cotton wool moistened with cool boiled water, working from the inner corner of the eye outwards. A fresh pad should be used on each eye, to limit infection. If the condition does not resolve after several days, allopathic advice should be sought.

- Neuralgic pains in the eyes, with flow of tears, from weakness or exhaustion after an illness.
  Kali phos 6x, a tissue salt, every 3–4 hours.
- Dry, inflamed, glaring eyes, pupils dilated, with absence of any discharge.
  Belladonna 6c, every 3–4 hours.
- Eyes inflamed, with swelling of the lids, pain, and occasional, hot, watery discharge. Patient anxious, restless, and feverish.
  Aconite 6c, every 3–4 hours.
- Eyes red and inflamed, with burning relieved by cold applications. Often resulting from overstrain. Patient nervous and sensitive.
  Ferrum phos 6x, a tissue salt, every 3–4 hours.
- Eyes inflamed, burning and watering, irritating discharge, patient cannot bear bright light.
  Euphrasia 6c, every 3–4 hours.
- Eyes red, painful and burning, particularly inside the eyelids, with acrid, burning discharge. Better from warm applications. Eyes can scarcely be opened.
  Arsenicum album 6c, every 3–4 hours.
- Pale, watery discharges, with puffy eyes, particularly the lower lid.
  Apis 6c, every 3–4 hours.
- Eyes red and inflamed, with discharge of watery mucus or flow of tears. Discharge irritates the skin, may cause small blisters to form.
  Nat mur 6x, a tissue salt, every 3–4 hours.
- Sore eyes, with discharge white or grayish–white, or specks of white matter on the lids.
  Kali mur 6x, a tissue salt, every 3–4 hours.
- Profuse discharge that is bland, white or yellow.
  Pulsatilla 6c, every 3–4 hours.
- Golden-yellow, creamy discharge, eyelids stuck together in the morning, creamy coating on the back of the tongue.
  Nat phos 6x, a tissue salt, every 3–4 hours.
- Inflamed eyes with swollen eyelids, white or yellow discharge.
  Argentum nit 6c every 3–4 hours.
- Thick yellow discharge, with styes, little boils or small hard lumps on the eyelids.
  Silicea 6x, a tissue salt, every 3–4 hours.
- Discharge yellow and sticky, eyes swollen and hard to open, patient feverish, with oily sweat.
  Mercurius 6c, every 3–4 hours.

Constipation

Constipation is having less than one bowel movement per day. It can often be improved by drinking more water, introducing oil, fiber and roughage into the diet, and reducing the intake of refined foods. The diet should include plenty of fresh fruit, green vegetables, green salads and whole grains.

Constipation has three main causes: inadequate lubrication of the bowel, irregular peristaltic action and irregular operation of the sphincters of the digestive tract. Inadequate lubrication causes a dry stool that is difficult to pass; irregular peristalsis results in incomplete movements; irregular sphincter operation causes constipation at irregular intervals. Often these three causes can be mixed together.

Straining at stool increases the risk of hemorrhoids, which can easily become chronic in established constipation. It is wise to treat only occasional episodes of constipation with laxatives; recurrent or chronic constipation, especially with blood in the stools, should not be treated with laxatives and should be assessed professionally.

TREATMENT

■ Constipation with heat in rectum, inflammation and fever.
Ferrum phos 6x, a tissue salt, every 3–4 hours.

■ Stool difficult to pass, with abdominal distension immediately after eating.
Lycopodium 6c, every 3–4 hours.

■ Obstinate retention of stool—irregular, hard, unsatisfactory.
Nat mur 6x, a tissue salt, every 3–4 hours.

■ Stool large, hard, and difficult to expel; may recede when partly expelled.
Silicea 6x, a tissue salt, every 3–4 hours.

■ Frequent and ineffectual desire to defecate, producing only a little at a time which relieves for a while. Particularly after abuse of laxatives.
Nux vomica 6c, every 3–4 hours.

■ Stool like sheep's dung, crumbles as if very dry.
Mag mur 6c, every 3–4 hours.

■ Habitual constipation, with heat, discomfort, large and painful stools.
Sulphur 6c, every 3–4 hours.

■ Alternate constipation and diarrhea, with irritability.
Nux vomica 6c, every 3–4 hours.

- Constipation with light-colored stool, white or grayish coating on the tongue.
  Kali mur 6x, a tissue salt, every 3–4 hours.
- Inability of muscles to expel stool, muscles weak and relaxed, especially with anal fissure.
  Calc fluor 6x, a tissue salt, every 3–4 hours.
- Alternating constipation and diarrhea with heat or burning.
  Sulphur 6c, every 3–4 hours.
- Hard knotty stool, with biliousness, or stool soft and difficult to expel. No urge to use the bowels. Must strain, and stool is unformed, soft and sticky, yet passes with difficulty.
  Alumina 6c, every 3–4 hours.
- Constipation of infants, with occasional attacks of diarrhea.
  Nat phos 6x, a tissue salt, every 3–4 hours.
- Constipation with hard, scanty stool, one session can last for hours, with severe burning in rectum and tendency to anal fissures.
  Nit ac 6c, every 3–4 hours.
- Chronic constipation, often no urge to go for many days. Stools are large, hard, dry and painful; sufferer often has severe headache.
  Bryonia 6c, every 3–4 hours.
- Constipation with excessive gas.
  Lycopodium 6c every 3–4 hours.

- Constipation with no desire for stool, alternating with loose stools or diarrhea. Foul-coated tongue, headache and hemorrhoids.
  Hydrastis 6c, every 3–4 hours.
- Frequent desire to defecate, but stool difficult, hard and dry, with burning.
  Sulphur 6c, every 3–4 hours.
- Feeling of ball in rectum.
  Sepia 6c, every 3–4 hours.
- Constipation with pains after stool.
  Sepia 6c, every 3–4 hours.
- No urge to defecate, but bowel is full.
  Lycopodium 6c, every 3–4 hours.
- Difficult expulsion, leaving a sensation of much soreness.
  Nat mur 6x, a tissue salt, every 3–4 hours.
- Sensation of constant pressing down, without much urging.
  Nat mur 6x, a tissue salt, every 3–4 hours.
- From inactivity of the rectum, with heat and headache.
  Veratrum album 6c, every 3–4 hours.
- Stools large: much straining until exhausted, with cold sweat.
  Veratrum album 6c, every 3–4 hours.
- Feels better when constipated.
  Calc carb 6c, every 3–4 hours.

Cough

Cough may be acute or chronic, and may be dry, spasmodic, or loose, with a variety of colors of mucus discharge. There are many remedies for cough in homeopathic treatment, and often the choice of the correct remedy needs a careful study of the symptoms. If the cough is part of a cold or influenza, those sections of this chapter should be read first. Chronic cough, cough that fails to improve, and cough that returns periodically need professional assistance. Cough with persistent blood in the sputum needs allopathic advice.

TREATMENT

Dry cough

■ Short, acute, painful cough, with sore lungs and no expectoration.
Ferrum phos 6x, a tissue salt, every 3–4 hours.

■ Dry, hard cough with anxiety and restlessness, worse in the evening.
Aconite 6c, every 3–4 hours.

■ Cough brought on by dry, cold winds, with anxiety, restlessness.
Aconite 6c, every 3–4 hours.

■ Dry ringing or barking cough, with fever, anxiety and restlessness.
Aconite 6c, every 3–4 hours.

■ Dry, barking or repetitive cough with a sudden onset, a flushed, congested face, and strong pulse; patient is restless and sweaty, but dislikes being uncovered.
Belladonna 6c, every 3–4 hours.

■ Cough dry and painful, patient must hold chest and head.
Bryonia 6c, every 3–4 hours.

■ Cough with difficult breathing and dry throat, worse from movement.
Bryonia 6c, every 3–4 hours.

■ Dry, tickling, irritating, hacking cough, with pronounced thirst.
Nat mur 6x, a tissue salt, every 3–4 hours.

■ Dry, wheezing, barking cough, beginning around midnight. Spongia is a remedy for croup.
Spongia 6c, every 3–4 hours.

■ Dry, fatiguing cough, seldom loose, always worse in morning.
Nux vomica 6c, every 3–4 hours.

■ Cough from every exposure to cold air, worse from drafts, better from warm rooms.
Hepar sulph 6c, every 3–4 hours.

■ Irritable, dry, tickling cough during sleep, does not waken.
Chamomilla 6c, every 3–4 hours.

■ Cough with burning in chest and difficult breathing; loss of voice.
Phosphorus 6c, every 3–4 hours.

- Constant dry, tickling cough, coming at night, and better from warm air or putting head under blankets.
  Rumex 6c, every 3–4 hours.

Spasmodic cough

- Sudden and suffocating cough, with congested face and inability to exhale, especially in infants. If a child it cannot nurse because of blocked nose.
  Sambucus 6c, every 3–4 hours.
- Retching and vomiting while coughing, with nausea, but cough is no better.
  Ipecac 6c, every 3–4 hours.
- Sudden spasmodic attacks, tickling and wheezing, worse lying down. Patient holds chest with hands while coughing; may whoop, gag and retch.
  Drosera 6c, every 3–4 hours.
- Racking cough at night with sore throat and thirst, greasy sweat.
  Mercurius 6c, every 3–4 hours.

- Dry, spasmodic, constricted cough, that may result in the vomiting of phlegm, but patient feels no better afterwards.
  Ipecac 6c, every 3–4 hours.
- Crowing cough, with spasms going on almost to the point of suffocation, sometimes with vomiting or convulsion, patient better from sipping hot water.
  Cuprum met 6c, every 3–4 hours.
- Paroxysms of coughing without expectoration, loud and noisy, like whooping cough, relieved by hot drinks.
  Mag phos 6x, a tissue salt, every 3–4 hours.

Cough with clear expectoration

- Cough with clear, watery mucus, sometimes tasting salty, or with excessive watery discharge from eyes or nose.
  Nat mur 6x, a tissue salt, every 3–4 hours.

Cough with white expectoration

- Hoarse cough, with thick white mucus rattling in bronchi that is difficult to cough up, with white- or gray-coated tongue.
  Kalu mur 6x, a tissue salt, every 3–4 hours.

Cough with yellow or yellow-green expectoration

- Dry and painful cough, with soreness or burning in the chest, later with a small amount of yellow sputum, occasionally streaked with blood. The cough is often worse in a sitting position.
  Ferrum phos 6x, a tissue salt, every 3–4 hours.

- Raucous, noisy and rattling cough, with yellowish mucus that is difficult to cough up, improved by humidifiers and vapour baths. There can be a thin, yellowish, nasal discharge.
  Hepar sulph 6c, every 3–4 hours.

- Cough dry at night and helped by being in the sitting position, and productive during the day. Sputum is thick, yellow, bland and not irritating.
  Pulsatilla 6c, every 3–4 hours.

- Cough with expectoration of slimy yellow or watery yellow mucus, worse in a warm room and the evening, better in the open air.
  Kali sulph 6x, a tissue salt, every 3–4 hours.

- Loose cough with yellow or green–yellow mucus, sometimes streaked with blood.
  Calc sulph 6x, a tissue salt, every 3–4 hours.

- Chronic cough with thick, profuse, yellowish–green mucus, always worse from cold drinks, in the morning on rising, or on lying down at night.
  Silicea 6x, a tissue salt, every 3–4 hours.

Loose and rattling cough

- Raucous cough, with rattling, wheezing and anxious breathing, even to the point of threatened suffocation.
  Hepar sulph 6c, every 3–4 hours.

- Moist hollow cough, much rattling in the chest, worse 4–8 p.m.
  Lycopodium 6c, every 3–4 hours.

- Loose cough, chest sore and painful; worse from damp.
  Nat sulph 6x, a tissue salt, every 3–4 hours.

- Wheezy chest with much thick mucus, rattling loudly but difficult to bring up. Worse 3–4 a.m., and better from sitting up.
  Ant tart 6c, every 3–4 hours.

Cramp

Cramp is muscle spasm, caused by interference with the nerve supply to the tissue, or the circulation. Useful treatments include massage of the affected part, applying hot compresses and checking for excessive losses of calcium, magnesium or salt. Abdominal cramps and chest cramps should always be viewed cautiously, and allopathic advice sought if appropriate remedies fail to improve cramps of any kind.

TREATMENT

- Cramps in any location, better from heat and pressure.
  Mag phos 6x, a tissue salt, every 3–4 hours, with a little hot water.
- Cramps in any location, feeling numb and cold, as if parts were asleep. Better from heat but not pressure.
  Calc phos 6x, a tissue salt, every 3–4 hours.
- Very acute pains with restlessness and irritability, may drive patient out of bed to pace about.
  Chamomilla 6c, every 3–4 hours.
- Abdominal cramps, running down the thighs.
  Chamomilla 6c, every 3–4 hours.

- Cramping pains radiate from abdomen to back, chest and arms, worse when bending double and while lying down, better by bending backwards.
  Dioscorea 6c, every 3–4 hours.
- Cramps in legs and arms of pregnant women.
  Viburnum op 6c, every 3–4 hours.
- Agonizing pain in abdomen, as if clamped by iron bands, forcing patient to bend double and apply hard pressure.
  Colocynth 6c, every 3–4 hours.
- Spasms and cramps in muscles in nape of neck, and spasmodic drawing back of the head. Back bends backwards, like an arch.
  Cicuta 6c, every 3–4 hours.

Cystitis

Cystitis is inflammation of the bladder, usually with painful, frequent urination. It can come on suddenly, with urgency, incontinence and spasm.

Urine may be passed in copious or minute amounts, and may be tinged with blood. Drink plenty of water and avoid acid fruits and fruit juices. Obstinate cystitis can indicate infection and a deeper disorder, and professional advice should be sought to avoid kidney infection.

TREATMENT

■ First stage of cystitis, with frequent urination and burning pain, or difficult and suppressed urination with constant urging.
Ferrum phos 6x, a tissue salt, every 3–4 hours.

■ Bladder painful, with violent cutting pains and great urging; intense burning pains before and after urination. Urine passed drop by drop with constant urging, extreme pain. Urine may be tinged with blood.
Cantharis 12c, every 4 hours.

■ Pain during and after urination, in copious amounts; great urge to urinate, with pain in the bladder as if full, but urination does not help much, so the patient must try again and again. Equisetum is useful in bedwetting in children.
Equisetum 6c, every 3–4 hours.

■ Ineffectual urging to urinate after or during intercourse, with pressure on the bladder and a feeling that it did not empty. Pain in the urethra when not urinating, that is better on passing urine. Often after or during intercourse and often in newly married women.
Staphysagria 6c, every 3–4 hours.

■ Constant desire to urinate, with sharp, stinging pains and increased volume of urine. No thirst.
Apis 6c, every 3–4 hours.

■ Pain in the urethra and bladder on urinating, extending into the thighs and hips. The small of the back and region of the kidneys feel bruised, stiff and lame. Fatigue, exercise, standing, any jarring movement, worsens the pain.
Berberis 6c, every 3–4 hours.

■ Frequent urination, with pain at the end—almost unbearable, and often accompanied by painful, spasmodic straining.
Sarsaparilla 6c, every 3–4 hours.

■ Urination intermittent and painful, with bloated abdomen and strong urging. The urine is red, brown, black or smoky in appearance, with burning and smarting.
Terebinth 6c, every 3–4 hours.

■ Painful urging, with small amounts of urine, dark or bloody.
Mercurius 6c, every 3–4 hours.

- Dark red urine containing thick, white mucus, and swelling of the tissues.
  Kali mur 6x, a tissue salt, every 3–4 hours.
- Cystitis with nervousness and debility. Scalding urine, with cutting pain.
  Kali phos 6x, a tissue salt, every 3–4 hours.
- Ineffectual and painful straining, urine passes in drops. Severe spasmodic pains. Constant urging to urinate when standing or walking.
  Mag phos 6x, a tissue salt, every 3–4 hours.
- Urethra swollen and inflamed, with frequent painful urination with cutting pain afterwards. Desire sudden and urgent, not easily controlled. There can be a sensation of trickling.
  Thuja 6c, every 3–4 hours.
- Kidney pain relieved after discharge of urine containing sand. Pain is worse on the right side—or begins on the right and moves to the left.
  Lycopodium 6c, every 3–4 hours.
- Profuse urination at night of clear watery urine, preceded by anxiety and followed by burning.
  Phosphoric acid 6c, every 3–4 hours.
- Urine is increased in volume, clear and watery, with pains just after urinating. There may be involuntary release during coughing, walking, or sneezing.
  Nat mur 6x, a tissue salt, every 3–4 hours.
- Intense sensation of burning, as if due to pepper in urine; urine is copious and clear.
  Capsicum 6c, every 3–4 hours.
- Intermittent flow of urine— flows and then stops again, even if bladder is not empty. May be also dribbling of urine.
  Conium 6c, every 3–4 hours.
- Cystitis after injury.
  Arnica 6c, every 3–4 hours.
- Must wait a long time to urinate.
  Arnica 6c, every 3–4 hours.
- Bladder is irritable, sensitive to jarring and pressure.
  Belladonna 6c, every 3–4 hours.

Diarrhea

Three or more loose movements per day is considered to be diarrhea. The movements are watery, and may contain mucus, undigested food or blood. The cause may be simple, such as dietary excess, or an episode of anxiety. In many cases it may be due to a temporarily inflamed colon, probably due to food that was not fresh or that did not suit.

If the colon is **irritable,** it is overactive but otherwise normal. There may be bouts of diarrhea, with or without pain. Bouts may be associated with emotional trauma, stress, or debility. If the colon is **spastic,** there is consistently more pain, caused by spasms of the colon. The pains are relieved by the passing of wind or stool. If the mucous membrane of the colon is disordered, **mucous colitis** can result. This can lead to bouts of diarrhea, often with the passing of large masses of mucus.

Ulcerated colon is usually accompanied by pain, fever and profuse diarrhea accompanied by blood and mucus, and should receive immediate allopathic attention.

Acute attacks of diarrhea that recur at intervals of weeks or months, or with accompanying fever of persistent blood in the stools, should be assessed professionally. Avoid dehydration in children and infants.

TREATMENT

■ Painless diarrhea with bitter taste, abdominal distension, rumbling and wind. Vomiting and great weakness; hunger but no appetite.
China 6c, every 3–4 hours.

■ Stool offensive, gushing, yellow and watery, worse in the early morning, with colicky pains. Better from heat and lying on abdomen.
Podophyllum 6c every 3–4 hours.

■ Diarrhea and vomiting with cold sweat, exhaustion and great coldness of skin, even collapse. Veratrum album is another good travellers' remedy.
Veratrum album 6c, every 3–4 hours.

■ Watery diarrhea, burning and stinging, with vomiting, exhaustion, restlessness and thirst for small drinks. Violent burning pains in the abdomen, improved by heat. Arsenicum is a good remedy in food poisoning and the diarrhea of travellers.
Arsenicum 6c, every 3–4 hours.

■ Diarrhea immediately after eating or drinking, with a great deal of wind and lack of confidence in the anal sphincter.
Aloes 6c, every 3–4 hours.

■ Diarrhea with painful cramps, starting and stopping suddenly, made better by doubling up, by heat and strong pressure.
Colocynthis 6c, every 3–4 hours.

- Diarrhea with white-coated tongue and variable stools, changeable in color and frequency. Much gas and rumbling, worse from fats and rich food.
  Pulsatilla 6c, every 3–4 hours.
- Diarrhea in spasms, with great nausea, not helped by vomiting. Stools offensive, yellow–green and frothy, sometimes bloody.
  Ipecac 6c, every 3–4 hours.
- Stools liquid but containing solid lumps, with belching of undigested food and a white tongue. Often after overeating, with nausea and vomiting, which do not improve.
  Ant crud 6c, every 3–4 hours.
- Loose movements driving patient out of bed every morning, with spasm of pain.
  Ignatia 6c, every 3–4 hours.
- Debility and weakness, with digestive disturbances, after long-continued diarrhea.
  China 6c, every 3–4 hours.
- Yellow, watery diarrhea, expelled in a jet like a pistol shot, worsened by even small amounts of food or drink. Often after antibiotics.
  Croton tig 6c, every 3–4 hours.
- Stool gushing like fire hydrant, with small lumps of white mucus, and with exhaustion.
  Phosphorus 6c, every 3–4 hours.
- Diarrhea at upredictable times, after emotional crisis.
  Ignatia 6c, every 3–4 hours.
- Stool yellow, offensive and urgent, driving patient out of bed in morning.
  Sulphur 6c, every 3–4 hours.
- Stool greenish like chopped spinach, with irritability and burning of the anus.
  Chamomilla 6c, every 3–4 hours.
- Stool greenish or clay-colored, offensive, may be bloody. Diarrhea is worse at night, with great straining, but always a sensation of incompleteness.
  Mercurius 6c, every 3–4 hours.

Earache

The common causes of earache include outer ear infection, where the pain is made worse by pulling on the lobe, middle ear infection or eustachian tube blockage, where the pain comes on suddenly, and a build-up of ear wax, where the pain comes on gradually. Another cause is pressure trauma after air travel, which gives a painful, blocked feeling not relieved by swallowing. Earache with pains in the jaw, teeth, face or throat may be caused by dental problems, sinusitis or a throat infection. Earache accompanied by a discharge of blood is usually a sign of an acute infection.

Ears should be treated with care and should not be poked. Any wax in the ear can be cleared by running warmed olive oil gently into the canal, until it is full. The oil should be kept in the ear for about ten minutes, then allowed to run out. Insects and other objects may also be cleared using this method. Do not attempt to clear wax during an infection.

Be cautious about the home homeopathic treatment of earache, as untreated infection can cause scarring and serious damage to the hearing. As a general rule, homeopathic treatment should only be used in uncomplicated earache, when there is inflammation but no evidence of discharge. In these cases, or when the earache is recurrent, the following remedies can be used while professional advice is being sought.

TREATMENT

■ Earache with fever, pain and congested face, or flushing, with alternate pallor and redness, occasionally with nosebleed.
Ferrum phos 6x, a tissue salt, every 30–60 minutes.

■ Earache with burning pain, coming on suddenly, with anxiety, irritability and restlessness.
Aconite 6c, every 30–60 minutes.

■ Earache with fever, heat and throbbing, patient flushed and restless. Worse from warmth, and sensitive to noise, movement and touch.
Belladonna 6c, every 30–60 minutes.

■ Earache with throbbing pains made better by warmth. Ear sensitive to cold and draughts, feels bruised and sore.
Hepar sulph 6c, every 1–2 hours.

■ Earache in restless, irritable types, driving patient to pace constantly.
Chamomilla 6c, every 30–60 minutes.

■ Earache with sharp neuralgic pains in or around the ear.
Mag phos 6x, a tissue salt, every 3–4 hours.

■ Pain as if pressure behind the eardrum is pushing it out. Person is irritable, changeable and restless, prefers open air.
Pulsatilla 6c, every 30–60 minutes.

- Earache with swelling of the glands and tongue coated white. **Kali mur 6x**, *a tissue salt, every 3–4 hours.*
- Earache with yellow catarrh of the ear and yellow tongue. **Kali sulph 6x**, *a tissue salt, every 3–4 hours.*
- Shooting pains in the ears. **Hypericum 6c**, *every 30–60 minutes.*
- Pain is stinging and burning, better by cold applications. **Apis 6c**, *every 30–60 minutes.*
- Patient is tearful and seeks comfort, but not irritable. Pain centres behind the ear, is sensitive to touch, and is made better by hot applications. **Capsicum 6c**, *every 30–60 minutes.*
- Deafness, with noises in the ear, from nervous weakness or exhaustion. **Kali phos 6x**, *a tissue salt, every 3–4 hours.*

Eczema

Eczema is a skin rash characterised by itching, swelling, thickening, scaling and blistering (dry eczema) or oozing, weeping and discharging (wet eczema). It is a common allergic reaction in children but it also occurs in adults, usually in more severe form. Childhood eczema often begins in infancy, the rash appearing on the face, neck and folds of elbows and knees, and is often due to an allergy to cow's milk or formula. It may disappear by itself when the offending food is removed from the diet, or it may become more extensive and in some instances cover the entire surface of the body.

Seborrheic eczema seems to be inherited, and not linked to an allergy. It shows as a flaking itchiness in the smile lines between the nose and mouth, in the beard area, around the hairline, in the scalp, groin and armpits, and on the chest. Severe eczema can be complicated by skin infections.

The orthodox treatment of eczema commonly involves the use of steroid ointments to relieve the inflammation, and sometimes antihistamines and antibiotics to control the itching and infection. The homeopathic treatment of eczema involves constitutional treatment; however, the following remedies can be used for general treatment. Steroid ointments should be avoided except in extreme cases.

- As a general application to help itching and drying in dry eczema.
  Chickweed ointment or *Urtica* tincture, *morning and evening.*
- In wet eczema.
  Chickweed ointment or *Calendula* tincture, *morning and evening.*
- Dry eczema in hot, sweaty types with rough, itching skin, made worse from washing and the heat of the bed.
  Sulphur 6c, morning and evening for several weeks. Stop and wait if there is a reaction.
- Dry, red areas often with small blisters, made better by warmth and worse in cold damp weather and at night. Usually on the hands, wrists and the bends in the joints.
  Rhus tox 6c, morning and evening for several weeks. Stop and wait if there is a reaction.

- Dry eczema, can be red and raised, cracked and bleed. Skin looks dirty, smells musty; itching is worse from warmth and the heat of the bed.
  Psorinum 6c, morning and evening for several weeks. Stop and wait if there is a reaction.
- Skin dry and itchy, also constipated.
  Alumina 6c, morning and evening for several weeks. Stop and wait if there is a reaction.
- Skin dry and burning, worse around midnight, made better by hot applications.
  Arsenicum 6c, morning and evening for several weeks. Stop and wait if there is a reaction.
- Wet eczema, oozing a clear or yellow honey-like discharge, often on the palms, behind the ears and on the head.
  Graphites 6c, morning and evening for several weeks. Stop and wait if there is a reaction.

Exhaustion, Debility and Fatigue

Fatigue, debility and exhaustion are all states of lowered vitality. They can spring from many causes, but notably a lack of sunshine, exercise, fresh air, sensible diet and positive mental attitude. Lowered vitality often occurs as the aftermath of an illness, especially one involving loss of vital fluids such as blood and digestive secretions. It is also seen as the result of the abuse of stimulants and from too little sleep. Supplementation of the diet with vitamins and minerals should always be thought of, but if the condition persists professional advice should be sought.

TREATMENT

- Nervous exhaustion after long-continued strain or intense study. Patient is easily irritable, excessively sensitive, even slight noises can prevent sleep.
  Kali phos 6x, a tissue salt, every 3–4 hours.

- Weakness after loss of blood and other vital fluids, especially with flatulence, diarrhea and other digestive disturbances.
  China 6c, every 3–4 hours.

- Vital forces nearly exhausted, cold, especially from knees to feet, with cold sweat on limbs. Starved for oxygen, asks for fresh air and to be fanned.
  Carbo veg 6c, every 3–4 hours.

- Fatigue with nerve pains, muscle cramps and twitching.
  Mag phos 6x, a tissue salt, every 3–4 hours.

- Low vitality, with lack of brain or nerve power. Fidgety feet. Aching and weariness in the nape of the neck as if it had been held in one position too long.
  Zincum 6c, every 3–4 hours.

- Great fatigue, with weakness and drowsiness. Sleepy and dull, cannot think clearly or fix attention. The legs and hands tremble, the eyelids droop.
  Gelsemium 6c, every 3–4 hours.

- Debility with great apathy and indifference, especially in stressed adults and in young people worn down by hard study.
  Phos ac 6c, every 3–4 hours.

- Great weakness and weariness, yet restless, especially midnight to 3 a.m. Exhaustion from the slightest exertion, patient craves heat and hot drinks.
  Arsenicum alb 6c, every 3–4 hours.

- Extreme exhaustion of mind and body, with great weakness in the chest, so weak patient is unable to talk. The weakness is worse from talking, laughing, reading aloud, singing. There is usually a loose cough.
  Stannum 6c, every 3–4 hours.

- Exhaustion and debility, especially in the old, with emaciation even though appetite and thirst may be excessive.
  Secale 6c, every 3–4 hours.

- Weakness and exhaustion in the elderly, sensitive to the cold, with offensive foot sweats.
  Baryta carb 6c, every 3–4 hours.
- Debility in women, from too much or too little work, with sensations of dragging and weight in the abdomen.
  Helonias 6c, every 3–4 hours.
- Debility with a strong sensation of internal trembling, though externally it is not visible. There is often a craving for wine or stimulants, especially after alcoholism.
  Sulph ac 6c, every 3–4 hours.
- Exhaustion with tired feeling all over the body, and accompanied by weakness of mind, indifference, want of will power and a desire to lie down. Even the slightest mental exertion may bring on a headache.
  Picric ac 6c, every 3–4 hours.
- Apathy, sluggishness and difficulty in speaking, patient restless and fearful.
  Phosphorus 6c, every 3–4 hours.
- Great weariness and debility, patient wants constantly to lie down.
  Silicea 6x, a tissue salt, every 3–4 hours.
- Great weakness, faintlike, with sinking of strength and trembling, drooping of the eyelids.
  Causticum 6c, every 3–4 hours.
- Depression with anemic paleness and emaciation, even though eating well.
  Nat mur 6x, a tissue salt, every 3–4 hours.
- To aid recovery after exhaustion, and promote the assimilation of nutrients.
  Calc phos 6x, a tissue salt, every 3–4 hours.

Fibrositis

Fibrositis is a popular term applied to muscular rheumatism. It is caused by small adhesions between muscle fibres, resulting in pain and stiffness. It is usually the result of habitual strain and emotional tension. It is one of the most common causes of backache.

TREATMENT

Avoid the use of mentholated creams and ointments while taking homeopathic remedies, as the remedies are neutralized by camphor and menthol.

- Acute, inflammatory pain, with redness and heat.
Ferrum phos 6x, a tissue salt, every 3–4 hours.
- Acute cramping pains, relieved by warmth.
Mag phos 6x, a tissue salt, every 3–4 hours.
- Pain coming on after unaccustomed strain, exercise or physical overwork, with bruised pain worse from movement.
Arnica 6c, every 3–4 hours.
- Stiffness and pain after exercise or overuse, worse on initial movement but better on limbering up and from heat.
Rhus tox 6c, every 3–4 hours.
- Pain from straining tendons, feels bruised and stiff, worse from cold and better from movement.
Ruta grav 6c, every 3–4 hours.

- Fibrositis in neck, back, and limbs, made worse by movement and better by stillness and pressure.
Bryonia 6c, every 3–4 hours.
- Stiffness and weakness in limbs, with aching, tearing pains, worse in cold weather and better in warm or humid weather.
Causticum 6c, every 3–4 hours.
- Pain and stiffness relieved by cold applications such as ice packs.
Ledum 6c, every 3–4 hours.
- Pain and stiffness coming on before a storm, becoming worse during rest and better from motion.
Rhododendron 6c, every 3–4 hours.
- Aching pain and stiffness, especially in the neck and shoulders, causing intense pain and spasm; feels as if patient must move, but movement worsens the pain.
Phytolacca 6c, every 3–4 hours.

Genital Herpes

Genital herpes is a viral disorder in the same family as cold sores. It is transmitted by oral–genital or genital–genital contact with someone who is incubating the virus, and shows as crops of small blisters, itching and burning, on the penis or vulva. They quickly become moist and ulcerated, often with swelling and tenderness of glands in the groin, and a mild fever appears. The symptoms usually clear within two weeks, but may recur periodically during stressful periods, when the health is below par, or when the immune system is weakened. Genital herpes in an expectant mother can be passed on to the child during birth, with risk of localisation in the baby's nervous system and the possibility of complications such as meningitis or encephalitis developing. In these cases a cesarean delivery must be employed to avoid infection.

TREATMENT

- As a general preventative.
  Herpes progenitalis nosode 30c,
  morning and evening for a few days.
- As a general treatment, as soon as irritation is felt or recurrence suspected.
  Borax 6c, every 3–4 hours.
- Small blisters, itching and burning, with restlessness.
  Rhus tox 6c, every 3–4 hours.
- Pearl-like blisters, hot and puffy, with dry skin.
  Nat mur 6x, a tissue salt, every 3–4 hours.

- Genitals burn and sting, with cracked skin and red, itchy rash.
  Capsicum 6c, every 3–4 hours.
- Itching lesions that form thick, yellow crusts.
  Petroleum 6c, every 3–4 hours.
- Ulcers that bleed, especially at night. Whole genital area tender and painful.
  Sempervivum 6c, every 3–4 hours.

Glandular Fever

Glandular fever is otherwise known as infectious mononucleosis, and is a viral disease affecting children, teenagers and adults. It most often occurs in adolescents and those passing through growth spurts, emotional stress or in other ways being at a low ebb. It begins as an influenza-type illness, with fatigue, headache and aching muscles, and is usually followed by a fever and swollen glands. There is often a sore throat that does not respond to antibiotics. A measles-like rash is common in the first two weeks; there may also be jaundice and abdominal pain later. The illness is infectious from just before the symptoms appear until the fever and sore throat are gone. Glandular fever can last from several weeks to many months. Episodes of debility, sweat and fever can occur sporadically during this time.

TREATMENT

- Lethargy, with weakness and drowsiness. Head and muscular pains, swollen or ulcerated throat. Enlarged glands, and blotchy rash.
  Ailanthus 6c, *every 3–4 hours.*
- As general protection for family and friends.
  Glandular fever nosode 30c, *once daily for 7 days.*

- Great sensation of coldness, with sore throat and chronic swelling of the glands. Rash of small, painful, itchy pimples.
  Cistus canadensis 6c, *every 3–4 hours.*

Hemorrhoids

Hemorrhoids are varicose veins in the rectum, and are otherwise known as piles. They are always present to some degree in patients prone to prolapse, but may occur as isolated episodes in almost anyone. Often they will come as a result of straining at stool, particularly during episodes of constipation, or as a result of dietary indiscretion. Hemorrhoids that appear for no apparent reason but do not improve, or which gradually enlarge and bleed, should receive professional assessment.

TREATMENT

- As a local application.
  Pilewort ointment or Hamamelis ointment, *applied to the affected area.*
- Sensation of dryness, burning and fullness of the rectum, with pains like needles.
  Aesculus 6c, *every 3–4 hours.*
- Itching hemorrhoids, painful some hours after stool, with constipation and irritability.
  Nux vomica 6c, *every 3–4 hours.*

- Hemorrhoids protruding like grapes, with scraped, burning sensation, made better by cold applications.
  Aloes 6c, *every 3–4 hours.*
- Sensitive hemorrhoids with bruised feeling, worse from the slightest touch—even the touch of toilet paper is painful.
  Mur ac 6c, *every 3–4 hours.*

- Burning, itching hemorrhoids, usually with constipation.
  Sulphur 6c, every 3–4 hours.
- Pain from hemorrhoids during and after a bowel motion, often with a fissure in the anus.
  Paeonia 6c, every 3–4 hours.
- Hemorrhoids inflamed and bleeding.
  Ferrum phos 6x, a tissue salt, every 3–4 hours.
- Hemorrhoids very tender and oozing dark blood.
  Hamamelis 6c, every 3–4 hours.
- Prolapsing, painful hemorrhoids, with shooting pains and abundant bleeding, improved by cold and sitting on a hard seat.
  Kali carb 6c, every 3–4 hours.
- Hemorrhoids that tend to bleed easily, in constipated cases where there is difficulty in passing large stool.
  Collinsonia 6c, every 3–4 hours.
- Hemorrhoids with severe itching and fissures of the anus.
  Graphites 6c, every 3–4 hours.
- During pregnancy and after birth, feeling bruised and swollen.
  Arnica 6c, every 3–4 hours.
- During pregnancy and after birth, with stinging.
  Apis 6c, every 3–4 hours.
- A longer-term constitutional treatment, to prevent return of hemorrhoids.
  Calc fluor 6x, a tissue salt, every 3–4 hours.

Hay Fever

Hay fever usually begins as irritation of the nasal membrane, with swelling, dryness, and tickling, culminating in episodes of sneezing. It is quickly followed by smarting, watery eyes, and watery nasal discharge. Symptoms may appear quite suddenly.

A more accurate term for hay fever is allergic rhinitis, as hay is not the only offender. Dusts, pollens from grasses, weeds, trees and flowers, as well as other factors such as fungal spores and animal hair, may also induce it. It may be seasonal or perennial.

Homeopathic treatment based on the hay fever symptoms alone will give relief but not cure, as the fault is usually an allergic response to unavoidable airborne irritants, and represents a deep-seated reactive pattern. The seasonal type is more easily treated, as the symptoms are more acute and more obvious. Perennial rhinitis is usually little helped by acute remedies; it is best treated by constitutional treatment from a homeopath.

TREATMENT

The symptomatic remedies can be divided into three categories, based on the locality of the irritation and the kind of discharge. They are:

■ local irritation
■ irritant discharge
■ non-irritant discharge

Local irritation of the eyes and nose

■ Extremely chilly, often with severe frontal headache or nosebleeds. Eyelids red, face mottled, frequent spasms of severe sneezing. Nose is either stuffed up or running freely, often itching inside. There is a peculiar numbness of the throat, where the patient tries to scratch the affected parts with the tongue. Very sensitive to smells, especially flowers and garlic.
Sabadilla 6c, every 3–4 hours.

■ Itching and tingling of the nose with violent sneezing.
Silicea 6x, a tissue salt, every 3–4 hours.

■ Profuse watery secretions, stinging and burning, with much sneezing. Intense dryness of the mucous membranes of the nose and pharynx, with raw, burning sensation, particularly at the back of the nose, as if it was being scratched. Like sabadilla, there is hypersensitivity to smells.
Sanguinaria 6c, every 3–4 hours.

■ For hay fever after exposure to the sun. Watery symptoms with sensation of itching and tingling in the nose.
Nat mur 6x, a tissue salt, every 3–4 hours.

Irritant discharge

■ Nose and eyes stream, sneezing is severe and increases in frequency, lips and nostrils become sore. Worse: indoors, mornings and in heat; better: in the open air.
Ammonium mur 6c, every 3–4 hours.

■ Acrid, watery discharge, irritating the upper lip and nostrils; with inability to smell. There is the impression that the nose is blocked, despite the running discharge.
Allium cepa 6c, every 3–4 hours.

- Sneezing is violent and painful, due to tickle inside nose not relieved by sneezing. Profuse, watery, corrosive nasal discharge, irritating the lip. Burning of eyes and nose is a prominent sensation. Worse: change in weather, cold, open air. Patient often wakes around midnight, irritable and restless.
  Arsenicum alb 6c, every 3–4 hours.
- Sneezing with prickling in the nose, causing patient to pinch nose or bore into nostrils. Nose is stuffed up, especially on the right side, but may be running profusely, with irritation to the nostrils. The throat is usually involved. The eye symptoms are usually not severe. Worse at night, particularly the sneezing.
  Arum triph 6c, every 3–4 hours.
- Sneezing in bouts, with irritant discharge from the nose and eyes, better in the open air.
  Naphthalinum 6c, every 3–4 hours.

Non-irritant discharge

- Chilly and irritable, always worse in morning. Face feels hot; nose stuffed up at night, streams in morning. Nose and eyes itch and burn, extending to larynx and trachea. Prolonged spells of sneezing. Worse: mornings and cold, open air.
  Nux vomica 6c, every 3–4 hours.

- Much sneezing, with bland discharge from the nose. Eyes are red and burning, discharge acrid and irritating. The throat is often involved, with a hard, dry cough. Worse: light, wind, indoors, lying down. Better: in the open air.
  Euphrasia 6c, every 3–4 hours.
- Face full and hot. Aching all over, limbs feel heavy. Violent sneezing with tingling of the nose, streams in morning with irritating discharge. Throat dry and burning; swallowing causes pain in the ears. Eyes feel hot and heavy. Worse: spring and humid weather.
  Gelsemium 6c, every 3–4 hours.
- Profuse watery discharges with sneezing, and spasmodic cough followed by sneezing.
  Badiaga 6c, every 3–4 hours.

- Constant sneezing; nose may be stuffed up or streaming. Eyes swell and water, alternating with streaming nose. Worse: open air and damp, becoming chilled when hot.
  Dulcamara 6c, every 3–4 hours.

- The discharges are bland, and yellow or yellow–green. The nose is dry and constricted at night, abundant discharge in the morning and during the day.

Although chilly, patients have a marked aversion to heat and a desire for the cold, and open air. *Pulsatilla 6c, every 3–4 hours.*

Headache

Most headaches are due to strain on the muscles of the neck or head, or congestion of the muscles that supply them. Patients with headache usually have other symptoms, so the treatment must include all the symptoms, including emotional states, rather than the headache symptoms alone. Some of the most frequent causes of headache are defective eyesight, spinal misalignment, constipation, anxiety and living at too high a pressure, all of which would require attention. Nevertheless, the remedies given here will have considerable success. Headaches that are chronic, or that become more frequent and intense, should be viewed seriously. Allopathic advice should be sought, and an osteopath or chiropractor consulted.

TREATMENT

- Headache comes on suddenly with feelings of anxiety or apprehension. Sensation as if there is a tight band around the skull, or the brain is being forced out of the head. *Aconite 6c, every 3–4 hours.*
- For congested, throbbing pain in the temples or over the eyes, with red face or bloodshot eyes, and vomiting of undigested food. *Ferrum phos 6x, a tissue salt, every 3–4 hours.*

- Throbbing, drumming, congestive pain, with enlarged pupils and glassy eyes, patient flushed and restless, headache worse in the sun or from sudden movement. *Belladonna 6c, every 3–4 hours.*
- Sudden bursting, throbbing, hammering pain, often after exposure to the hot sun. *Glonoine 6c, every 3–4 hours.*
- Bursting, throbbing headache, improved by nosebleed or onset of menstrual bleeding. *Melilotus 6c, every 3–4 hours.*

■ Stinging, stabbing or burning headache, rest of the body feels bruised and tender. There is usually no thirst, and the symptoms are worse in hot, stuffy surroundings.
Apis 6c, every 3–4 hours.

■ Headaches from nervous tension, with piercing frontal pain and neck tension in zealous, irritable types, who suffer from insomnia.
Nux vomica 6c, every 3–4 hours.

■ Headache with dull, congestive, hammering pain, patient feels heavy and stupefied. May feel like there is a band around the head, with trembling of the hands and shivers up the spine.
Gelsemium 6c, every 3–4 hours.

■ After excessive alcohol or rich food, irritable and oversensitive, worse in morning. Nux vomica is the hangover remedy.
Nux vomica 6c, every 3–4 hours.

■ Dull, heavy headache, with profusion of tears, watery discharge from the nose or profuse saliva, frequently associated with constipation.
Nat mur 6x, a tissue salt, every 3–4 hours.

■ Headache from exhaustion, with apathy and inability to think or reflect. After severe debilitating illness, overwork, or in children who are growing too rapidly.
Phos ac 6c, every 3–4 hours.

■ Headaches of purely nervous character, from overstrain of the mental faculties, worry, sleeplessness or stress, in schoolchildren, students and overworked intellectuals.
Kali phos 6x, a tissue salt, every 3–4 hours.

■ Student's headaches; inability for thought, better from cheerful excitement or gentle motion.
Kali phos 6x, a tissue salt, every 3–4 hours.

■ Neuralgic headaches: excruciating, stinging, darting pain. Heat and pressure relieves, cold aggravates.
Mag phos 6x, a tissue salt, every 3–4 hours.

■ Sick headaches, with giddiness and dullness, bitter taste, greenish–gray coated tongue.
Nat sulph 6x, a tissue salt, every 3–4 hours.

■ Headache with white-coated tongue, or vomiting and hawking of white mucus.
Kali mur 6x, a tissue salt, every 3–4 hours.

■ Headache or migraine that often comes periodically, such as on Sundays or holidays with profuse vomiting that is acrid and burning.
Iris vers 6c, every 3–4 hours.

■ Headaches with sparks before the eyes.
Mag phos 6x, a tissue salt, every 3–4 hours.

- Migraine with pain under the eyes, especially the right side, accompanied by yellowish vomit, thick and sticky.
  Kali bich 6c, *every 3–4 hours.*
- Migraine or headache, with pain starting in the forehead and ending in the back of the head, with constipation.
  Lac deflor 6c, *every 3–4 hours.*
- Migraine worse from vibration, such as a lot of noise or talk, beginning each time on the opposite side, or starting at the base of the skull and settling over one eye.
  Lac caninum 6c, *every 3–4 hours.*
- Periodic migraine, coming on every 7 days, affecting especially the left side, beginning in the morning and worse from smells, noise, light and movement. Pains start at base of skull and extend over head to right eye.
  Sanguinaria 6c, *every 3–4 hours.*
- Hammering headache, preceded by misty vision or zig-zag lights.
  Nat mur 6x, *a tissue salt, every 3–4 hours.*
- Headache from eyestrain or from close application to fine work.
  Ruta grav 6c, *every 3–4 hours.*
- Headache with offensive taste in mouth, bad breath, worse at night and in the morning.
  Mercurius 6c, *every 3–4 hours.*
- Headache with painful, watering eyes, intolerance of bright light.
  Euphrasia 6c, *every 3–4 hours.*
- Headache with dry mouth and bruised, sharp, stabbing pain, made better by pressure and worse by the slightest motion; patient must lie still, with room dark and quiet.
  Bryonia 6c, *every 3–4 hours.*
- Headaches with a cold feeling in the head, or with creeping numbness and pain.
  Calc phos 6x, *a tissue salt, every 3–4 hours.*
- From overwork or emotional distress, in tearful types, better in the open air.
  Pulsatilla 6c, *every 3–4 hours.*
- Headaches of young girls with irregular menstruation and watery discharges.
  Nat mur 6x, *a tissue salt, every 3–4 hours.*
- Pain beginning in the neck, coming over the head, and ending in one eye.
  Silicea 6x, *a tissue salt, every 3–4 hours.*
- Bruised pain, especially after a blow.
  Arnica 6c, *every 3–4 hours.*
- Headache on the crown of the head, with acid, sour regurgitations, creamy-coated tongue.
  Nat phos 6x, *a tissue salt, every 3–4 hours.*

- Headache with wandering or changeable pain.
  Pulsatilla 6c, *every 3–4 hours.*
- As if temples were being screwed together.
  Lycopodium 6c, *every 3–4 hours.*
- With burning on top of head.
  Sulphur 6c, *every 3–4 hours.*

- Worse 4–8 p.m.
  Lycopodium 6c, *every 3–4 hours.*
- Worse from jarring, lying down.
  Belladonna 6c, *every 3–4 hours.*
- Pain reduced by bending head backwards.
  Hypericum 6c, *every 3–4 hours.*

Heart Pain

Heart pain is otherwise known as angina, and is a dull constricting pain felt in the centre of the chest, radiating up into the neck and jaw, and usually down the left arm. It is caused by restriction of the supply of blood and oxygen to the heart. Other symptoms can be dizziness, nausea, sweating and difficult breathing. If you suspect you are suffering from angina you should go to an allopath for a thorough checkup.

Unlike the pain of a heart attack, angina is often directly associated with excitement, exertion and stress, and will wear off after the excitement or exertion ceases. Nevertheless, angina can precede a full-blown heart attack, so if the pains do not wear off after five minutes, or become more severe, allopathic advice should be sought immediately. Constitutional homeopathic treatment is recommended.

TREATMENT

Treatment includes losing weight, taking daily moderate exercise, reducing stress, giving up smoking, avoiding animal fats, coffee and alcohol. Supplementation with fish oil and garlic is beneficial. Supplementation with vitamin E is also beneficial over the longer term, but must be started slowly.

- Pain and stitches in the heart region, as if squeezed, particularly after strain or exertion, with irregular pulse.
  Arnica 6c, *every 15 minutes in the acute case, and morning and evening over the longer term.*

- Sensation as if a band were constricting the chest or heart, with cold sweat, difficult breathing and pain down the left arm. Worse by lying on left side.
  Cactus grand 6c, *every 15 minutes for a few doses in the acute case, and morning and evening over the longer term.*

- Stitching pains, violent palpitations and difficult breathing, with thirst for hot water, person cannot bear to be touched. Symptoms are relieved by lying down on the right side with the head raised.
  Spigelia 6c *every 15 minutes for a few doses in the acute case, and morning and evening over the longer term.*

- Dull, pressing pain extending down the right arm with whole body pulsing, worse in a warm room.
  Lilium 6c *every 15 minutes for a few doses in the acute case, and morning and evening over the longer term.*

- Angina with irregular pulse, heart feels as if it has a weight on it, sensations of blood surging into the head, made worse by stimulants.
  Naja 6c, *every 15 minutes for a few doses in the acute case, and morning and evening over the longer term.*

- Angina with fluttering heart and sensation of pounding throughout the body. Person feels faint, with difficult breathing, worse by heat.
  Glonoine 6c, *every 15 minutes for a few doses in the acute case, and morning and evening over the longer term.*

- Violent chest pains, numbness in the fingers, feeble but rapid pulse.
  Latrodectus 6c, *every 15 minutes for a few doses in the acute case, and morning and evening over the longer term.*

- Stitching pains in the heart, can come at any time, bringing cries of pain. Person leans forward, resting on arms, to take the weight off the chest.
  Kali carb 6c, *every 15 minutes for a few doses in the acute case, and morning and evening over the longer term.*

- Congestion and anguish about the heart, with depression and melancholy. Great difficulty in breathing, person must lie down.
  Aurum 6c, *every 15 minutes for a few doses in the acute case, and morning and evening over the longer term.*

Heat Exhaustion

Heat exhaustion is caused by excessive fluid and salt loss in hot or humid conditions due to prolonged sweating, leading to general dehydration and exhaustion. Diarrhea and vomiting can also be predisposing causes. A person developing heat exhaustion shows symptoms of headache, excessive sweating, dizziness and weakness, with mild nausea. There may be fast, shallow breathing, cramps and muscle twitches, and a weak but rapid pulse. The temperature may be normal or below normal. Heat exhaustion shows symptoms similar to sunstroke; both have headache, dizziness and weakness, but in heat exhaustion there is sweating with a normal or below normal temperature, while in sunstroke there is a high temperature and absence of sweating. If the condition is unstable, or the patient collapses, allopathic attention is necessary.

TREATMENT

General treatment should include giving a little water to drink, with half a teaspoon of salt added per half-liter of water. The patient should lie down, with the legs elevated. The following remedies can be used in stable cases.

- Sudden drop in temperature, with red, dry skin and no sweat. Intense thirst, with high anxiety about condition.
  Aconite 6c, every 30 minutes.
- Throbbing, bursting headache, hot face and sweaty skin.
  Glonoine 30c, every hour.
- Fever with prostration, trembling and a crimson face. Severe headache radiating into the shoulders. Occasionally there are visual disturbances.
  Gelsemium 6c, every hour.

- Bright red face, and often with fluctuating temperature. Throbbing headache. Pulse strong and rapid; pupils fixed and dilated. Sensitive to noise, light and movement.
  Belladonna 6c, every 30–60 minutes.
- Headache, usually at the front, with oily sweat and intense thirst. Pain is worse on the slightest movement.
  Bryonia 6c, every 1–2 hours.
- When muscle cramps predominate.
  Cuprum met 6c, every 30–60 minutes

- Severe headache, with red congested face and rolling of the head from side to side. No thirst, and the skin is alternately dry, then moist with sweat.
  Apis 6c, every 15 minutes.
- Flushed face and congestive, throbbing headache, throbbing of arteries of head and neck, eyes red and bloodshot. Improved by appearance of bloody nose.
  Melilotus 6c, every 15 minutes..

Hives

Hives are properly known as **urticaria**, and can follow stings and trauma from plants such as nettles, although they are usually caused by allergic reaction to foods, medication or external pollutants. Hives may also be associated with worm infestations. They appear as intensely itchy red spots, in clusters or spread apart, and can occur anywhere. They may show as a fine rash or as well-defined, raised swellings.

TREATMENT

- As a local application.
  Tincture of urtica, or urtica cream, applied to the lesions.
- With feverish symptoms and anxiety, on first appearing.
  Aconite 6c, every 3–4 hours.
- With stinging pains and swelling, made worse from heat. Face and eyelids puffy.
  Apis 6c, every 3–4 hours.
- Burning, stinging rash and intense, intolerable itching, patient cannot refrain from scratching, has blotched and swollen face.
  Urtica 6c, every 3–4 hours.
- Small blisters or swollen rash, intensely itching and tingling, surrounded by red and swollen areas, with restlessness.
  Rhus tox 6c, every 3–4 hours.
- Eruptions are clear and watery, often from insect bites or after becoming overheated.
  Nat mur 6x, a tissue salt, every 3–4 hours.
- Feverish symptoms, dry and flushed.
  Ferrum phos 6x, a tissue salt, every 3–4 hours.
- With severe headache, hot and red face.
  Belladonna 6c, every 3–4 hours.

- Hives with dry skin, tending to scale.
  Kali sulph 6x, a tissue salt, every 3–4 hours.
- Hives with soreness of the skin and a creamy tongue.
  Nat phos 6x, a tissue salt, every 3–4 hours.
- Dry, burning, itching rash, worse from heat or hot water.
  Sulphur 6c, every 3–4 hours.
- Hives from eating shellfish.
  Camphor 6c, every 3–4 hours.
- Brought on by eating meat.
  Ruta grav 6c, every 3–4 hours.
- With burning and itching skin, often with gastric disorders, with white-coated tongue. Worse from warmth and the heat of the bed, worse on cheeks and chin.
  Ant crud 6c, every 3–4 hours.
- In chronic cases.
  Sulph ac 6c, every 3–4 hours.

Hoarseness and Loss of Voice

Hoarseness is caused by inflammation or infection of the larynx or vocal cords. It is commonly due to shouting or straining the voice, heavy smoking, or from a cold, sore throat or cough. Loss of voice is more commonly caused by vocal overuse than by infection.

TREATMENT

- Hoarseness caused by overuse of the voice, such as singing, shouting or screaming. Sudden loss of voice.
  Arnica 6c, every 3–4 hours.
- Painful hoarseness of speakers and singers due to strain of the vocal cords or from catching cold.
  Ferrum phos 6x, a tissue salt, every 3–4 hours.
- Hoarseness with raw, dry throat, that is hard to clear or swallow, and a scraping or burning sensation. Desire for cold drinks.
  Causticum 6c, every 3–4 hours.
- Hoarseness at the beginning of speaking, improving from continued use.
  Rhus tox 6c, every 3–4 hours.

- Hoarseness with itchy, painful larynx, made worse from speaking, and that brings on a hard, dry cough and loss of voice.
  Phosphorus 6c, every 2–3 hours.
- Hoarseness worse during menstruation.
  Gelsemium 6c, every 3–4 hours.
- Hoarseness with swollen, burning throat and loss of voice. Voice difficult to control, pitch varies, and voice worse from use.
  Arum triph 6c, every 3–4 hours.
- Voice feeble due to overuse, with tickle in the larynx made worse by cold.
  Alumina 6c, every 3–4 hours.
- Voice weak and trembling, inclined to break, with tickle in the larynx.
  Argentum met 6c, every 3–4 hours.
- Loss of voice with croup or a dry, barking cough.
  Spongia 6c, every 3–4 hours.
- Loss of voice from cold. Croupy cough, with abundant white mucus, and a white-coated tongue.
  Kali mur 6x, a tissue salt, every 3–4 hours.
- Chronic hoarseness with much clearing and scraping of the throat.
  Calc phos 6x, a tissue salt, every 3–4 hours.
- Loss of voice from paralysis of the vocal cords.
  Oxalic acid 6c, every 3–4 hours.
- Hysterical loss of voice.
  Ignatia 6c, every 3–4 hours.
- Chronic loss of voice without obvious cause.
  Baryta carb 6c, every 3–4 hours.
- Laryngitis with barking cough and tickling, dry throat.
  Drosera 6c, every 2–3 hours.

Incontinence of Urine

Incontinence of urine often occurs in the elderly, usually through loss of control of the bladder sphincters, and less often because of spinal problems, or brain damage after a stroke. Stress incontinence—momentary loss of control when laughing, coughing, etc.—is primarily a female problem and is due to weakness of the pelvic floor muscles. Involuntary dribbling after the end of urination in men is often a prostate disorder, which should be checked by an allopath.

■ Incontinence due to weakness of sphincter, with pain in the neck of the bladder, aggravated by standing, relieved by urinating. *Ferrum phos 6x*, a tissue salt, every 3–4 hours.

■ Incontinence from nervous weakness. *Kali phos 6x*, a tissue salt, every 3–4 hours.

■ Incontinence because of paralysis of the bladder muscles, with weak, trembly legs. *Gelsemium 6c*, every 3–4 hours.

■ Involuntary urination when walking or coughing. *Nat mur 6x*, a tissue salt, every 3–4 hours.

■ Incontinence made worse by coughing or laughing. *Causticum 6c*, every 3–4 hours.

■ Involuntary dribbling of urine after urination, especially in irritable men. *Nux vomica 6c*, every 3–4 hours.

Indigestion and Heartburn

Indigestion may be simply a sensation of discomfort after food, or marked by symptoms of nausea, heartburn, stomach congestion, wind and occasional vomiting as a result of faulty habits of eating. Particular habits to watch are eating too fast, eating too much, eating when not hungry, eating when tense or emotionally upset and excessive intake of rich food or alcohol. Treatment includes giving the digestion as much rest as possible by adopting regular eating habits, and selecting wholesome, easily digestible foods. Avoid late-night eating, and reduce coffee, tea and alcohol consumption. Try to stop smoking. Persistent pain or burning in the digestive tract may indicate ulcers or other problems and warrants allopathic examination.

TREATMENT

■ Stomach pain, tenderness and swelling, with a hot, flushed face and clean tongue. *Ferrum phos 6x*, a tissue salt, every 3–4 hours.

■ Spasmodic pains and cramp of the stomach, relieved by hot drinks. *Mag phos 6x*, a tissue salt, every 3–4 hours.

- Indigestion with sour risings and heartburn after eating. The tongue is creamy yellow at the back. Nat phos is a good remedy for simple acidity.
Nat phos 6x, a tissue salt. Can be used every 5 minutes in acute acidity, every 3–4 hours in the normal case.
- Indigestion, with discomfort, bloating and pain, especially in children and stressed adults.
Chamomilla 6c, every 3–4 hours.
- Indigestion several hours after eating. Food sits like a stone in the stomach with feeling of pressure under the breastbone, particularly from fats and rich foods. Patient feels worse in the evening. Creamy tongue and no thirst.
Pulsatilla 6c, every 3–4 hours.
- Indigestion from overloading the stomach, especially with fatty food, and thickly coated white tongue. Loss of appetite, nausea, distress. Feels as if must vomit for relief.
Ant crud 6c, every 3–4 hours.
- Indigestion after taking rich or fatty foods, with a whitish coating on the tongue.
Kali mur 6x, a tissue salt, every 3–4 hours.
- Indigestion every 1–2 hours after meals, improved by eating.
Anacardium 6c, every 3–4 hours.
- Nervous indigestion, with an empty, "gone" feeling in the stomach, often after fright or excitement.
Kali phos 6x, a tissue salt, every 3–4 hours.
- Digestive powers gradually weakening: patient irritable, pale and sallow. Frequent bloating after only a few mouthfuls. May be able to take only small meals.
Lycopodium 6c, every 3–4 hours.
- Much wind and flatulence, somewhat relieved by belching, in chilly persons who like fresh air. Digestion seems slower than usual, and the plainest food disagrees, especially fats. Often after weakening of the digestion by abuse of rich foods.
Carbo veg 6c, every 3–4 hours.
- Discomfort, nausea and flatulence every 30–60 minutes after eating or drinking alcohol, with irritability and sour, bitter belching.
Nux vomica 6c, every 3–4 hours.
- Flatulence, with uncomfortable distension of the whole abdomen, not relieved by belching. Person sluggish and apathetic, often after excessive loss of body fluids.
China 6c, every 3–4 hours.

- Bloating and flatulence after even a light meal, not relieved by belching; must loosen clothing. Much rumbling and gurgling in lower abdomen pressing downward, pain on right side and intolerance of fats.
Lycopodium 6c, every 3–4 hours.
- Flatulence with tenderness over the liver, craving pickles and acid foods, with sudden empty feeling in the stomach yet nauseated by the smell of food.
Sepia 6c, every 3–4 hours.
- Simple heartburn with excessive belching, may have nausea and fluttery feeling in stomach. Eating relieves the nausea, but makes the stomach worse. Improved by sour foods, but craves sweet foods, that disagree.
Argentum nit 6c, every 3–4 hours.
- Heartburn and discomfort, felt 30–60 minutes after eating in tense, irritable types. May have painful retching, leaving putrid taste in the mouth.
Nux vomica 6c, every 3–4 hours.
- Food lies like a stone in the stomach, with heartburn and bitter risings. Worse from pressure and movement, better while resting.
Bryonia 6c, every 3–4 hours.
- Burning sensation in the chest, with nausea and craving for ice cream or ice-cold water: may vomit.
Phosphorus 6c, every 3–4 hours.
- Heartburn often around midnight, stomach burning and heavy, person may retch and vomit till exhausted, better from warmth and small sips of water.
Arsenicum alb 6c, every 3–4 hours.
- Burning hunger pains, relieved by food and hot milk, but soon followed by indigestion. Nauseated by sweet things.
Graphites 6c, every 3–4 hours.
- Burning sensation in the stomach and the length of the bowel. Much thirst, but drinking causes shuddering.
Capsicum 6c, every 3–4 hours.
- Gastric disturbances with bilious symptoms, bitter taste in the mouth and vomiting of bitter fluids. The tongue may be coated greenish-brown or greenish-gray.
Nat sulph 6x, a tissue salt, every 3–4 hours.
- Gastric catarrh with slimy, golden–yellow coating of the tongue. Colicky pains in the stomach, with feeling of pressure and fullness.
Kali sulph 6x, a tissue salt, every 3–4 hours.
- Craves coffee, acids, sweet and salt things.
Carbo veg 6c, every 3–4 hours.
- Digestion seems very slow, especially after illness.
China 6c, every 3–4 hours.

- Long history of indigestion, with alternating constipation and diarrhea.
  Sulphur 6c, *every 3–4 hours.*

- To improve digestion and assimilation.
  Calc phos 6x, *a tissue salt, every 3–4 hours.*

Influenza

Influenza is a highly infectious disease, associated with a number of viruses. It often has symptoms very similar to those of colds, such as sneezing and streaming eyes, but influenza is more widespread in its symptoms: it usually begins with a sudden fever of short duration, with headache, prostration, severe pain in the body, chill and lassitude. Aches and pains in the bones and joints are prominent. Inflammation of the respiratory passages follows, with sneezing, cough, catarrh and hoarseness.

PREVENTION
Aconite, Belladonna, Gelsemium and Ferrum phos can be used in the early feverish stages of influenza, and will often stop the influenza progressing if given early enough. In addition, one homeopathic remedy, **Oscillococcinum 200c,** has a useful clinical anti-viral action, and can be obtained from a practitioner. It is given as one dose per week during the winter months, as a preventative of influenza. It is also useful when given as soon as the first symptoms appear, and the earlier it is given the more effective it is. Give one dose daily for one week. Taken later in the illness, it can usefully complement the action of the remedies given here.

TREATMENT

First stage
- In the first stage, with chills followed gradually by heat, fever, headache and vomiting.
  Ferrum phos 6x, *a tissue salt, every 3–4 hours.*
- May have a hard dry cough.
  Aconite 6c, *every 3–4 hours.*

- Flushed, restless, with pounding pulse and throbbing throughout the body. Violent headache. Usually there is no thirst.
  Belladonna 6c, *every 3–4 hours.*

- Influenza beginning with clear discharge from the eyes and nose. The throat is dry; thirst may be intense or absent. Much sneezing.
Nat mur 6x, a tissue salt, every 3–4 hours.

Established stage

- Intense bone pain: often the eye sockets and shins ache most intensely. Patient depressed, complains loudly and incessantly restless. There is an intensely dry throat, with thirst for ice-cold drinks, but sometimes no thirst at all.
Eupatorium 6c, every 3–4 hours.

- Pain through the whole body: wants to lie still and be left alone, and irritable if disturbed. Sweat is hot and considerable; cough, if present, is hard, dry and painful. The mouth is very dry, with thirst for large amounts of cold water. All pains are worse from movement.
Bryonia 6c, every 3–4 hours.

- Restless, yet weak and easily exhausted; irritable, wants to sit up. Great heat and burning in the chest, yet desires heat and hot drinks. Abundant discharge from the nose, thin and irritating. Breath short and difficult.
Arsenicum alb 6c, every 3–4 hours.

- Discharges are thick and white, with sore throat and a white-coated tongue. In the early stages, in alternation with Ferrum phos.
Kali mur 6x, a tissue salt, every 3–4 hours.

- Intense weariness, with dullness. Congested, slightly flushed with heavy eyelids. Usually no thirst. Comfortable propped up with pillows and lying still.
Gelsemium 6c, every 3–4 hours.

- Craves heat, yet cannot get warm enough; hugs the fire. Shivering and chilly, with violent cough. Worse from open air and especially after drinking, with chills as if blood turned to iced water.
Nux vomica 6c, every 3–4 hours.

- Fever progresses slowly, with increasing aching. Pain with great restlessness, has relief only in constant movement. Sweat is profuse and sour, with intensely dry mouth and lips; person takes small sips of water to keep the mouth moist. Cold sores often develop on the lower lip within 12 hours of onset of illness.
Rhus tox 6c, every 3–4 hours.

- Thick yellow discharges, with dry skin and desire for fresh air.
Kali sulph 6x, every 3–4 hours.

- Influenza with oily sweat, offensive mouth and breath. Thirsty, in spite of a sticky, fairly profuse salivation, and wants cold drinks. There is often conjunctivitis, with profuse, hot, irritating tears. Patient is uncomfortable all night, made worse by the heat of the bed, with a marked rise in temperature, and is liable to greasy sweats that bring no relief.
  Mercurius 6c, *every 3–4 hours.*
- For debility and weakness after influenza, to help convalescence and build up the constitution.
  Calc phos 6x, *a tissue salt, every 3–4 hours.*

Insomnia

The causes of insomnia in children are usually overexcitement and overstimulation, and remedies for them are in Chapter 5. In adults the causes are more diverse, but often center around an overactive mind, abuse of food, alcohol or coffee, or as the aftermath of stress.

TREATMENT

- Anxiety and fear, tossing about restlessly. Nightmares; cannot sleep. Sometimes after shock.
  Aconite 6c, *every 1–2 hours.*
- Insomnia following excitement, or from overwork, mental or physical. Can be excited or exhausted.
  Kali phos 6x, *a tissue salt, every 3–4 hours.*
- Insomnia after fright or shock.
  Aconite 6c, *every 3–4 hours.*
- Insomnia following grief, disappointed love, or other emotional shock.
  Ignatia 6c, *every 3–4 hours.*
- Insomnia around 3 a.m. until around dawn, from mental stress or too much study. Irritable that sleep will not come, especially after abuse of alcohol or coffee.
  Nux vomica 6c, *every 3–4 hours.*
- Insomnia from nervous stress and tension. Spells of yawning.
  Mag phos 6x, *a tissue salt, every 3–4 hours.*
- Mind overactive: cannot stop train of thought and flow of ideas.
  Coffea 6c, *every 3–4 hours.*

- Excessive sleep or constant desire to sleep, yet sleep is unrefreshing. Restless sleep, with constant starting.
  Nat mur 6x, a tissue salt, every 3–4 hours.
- Insomnia from oversensitivity to pain, drives out of bed to move about restlessly.
  Chamomilla 6c, every 3–4 hours.
- Sleepless from feverish congestions. Drowsy in the afternoon but unable to sleep at night.
  Ferum phos 6x, a tissue salt, every 3–4 hours.
- Can sleep in short naps only, then person wakes feeling unrefreshed.
  Phosphorus 6c, every 3–4 hours.
- Insomnia after exertion and physical strain, bed feels too hard.
  Arnica 6c, every 3–4 hours.
- Sleepy but cannot get to sleep.
  Chamomilla 6c, every 2–3 hours.
- Drowsy during the day, yet sleepless at night. Can get short naps only.
  Sulphur 6c, every 3–4 hours.
- Restless between midnight and 3 a.m., walks about, cannot relax, even though exhausted.
  Arsenicum 6c, every 3–4 hours.
- Drowsy and sleepy during the day, with bilious symptoms and gray–green tongue.
  Nat sulph 6x, a tissue salt, every 3–4 hours.
- Insomnia after overeating.
  Pulsatilla 6c, every 3–4 hours.
- Insomnia with itching of skin, burning of feet.
  Sulphur 6c, every 3–4 hours.
- Sleepless due to digestive disturbances and sour regurgitations.
  Nat phos 6x, a tissue salt, every 3–4 hours.

Jaundice

Jaundice is yellowness of the skin and whites of the eyes following the accumulation of bile products in the blood. It is usually due to poor liver function, although it can also arise from disorders such as blocked bile ducts in the gallbladder, or when blood cells break up due to haemolytic anemia. It may also arise from chemical poisons or drug prescription. It is a common symptom in newborn infants. Jaundice that comes on suddenly, with nausea and lethargy, should be assessed medically to make sure it is not infectious.

- Jaundice with a pain under right shoulder blade, a bitter taste, thickly coated tongue, loss of appetite, and nausea relieved by drinking hot water.
  Chelidonium 6c, every 3–4 hours.
- Early stages of jaundice, with inflammation, fever, pain in the liver and vomiting of undigested food.
  Ferrum phos 6x, a tissue salt, every 3–4 hours.
- Jaundice from congestion of the liver and gallbladder, with biliousness, flatulence and greenish stools.
  Nat sulph 6x, a tissue salt, every 3–4 hours.
- Jaundice with enlarged liver, constipation and clay-colored stools.
  Chionanthus 6c, every 3–4 hours.
- Yellow skin with great itching, worse at night and from the warmth of the bed. Tongue is large and flabby, showing the imprint of the teeth, and the breath is foul.
  Mercurius 6c, every 3–4 hours.

- Jaundice from abuse of rich food and alcohol, irritable, constipated and chilly.
  Nux vomica 6c, every 3–4 hours.
- Jaundice with empty, gnawing hunger, constipation, a dragging down feeling in the abdomen and indifference to loved ones.
  Sepia 6c, every 3–4 hours.
- Jaundice with swollen, hard liver, painful to touch. Bitter taste in the mouth and great bloating of the abdomen.
  China 6c, every 3–4 hours.
- Jaundice caused by a fit of anger.
  Chamomilla 6c, every 3–4 hours.
- Jaundice with light-colored stools, a white-coated tongue and a bitter taste.
  Kali mur 6x, a tissue salt, every 3–4 hours.
- Jaundice with pressure in the liver, sore and sensitive to motion and touch. Even a deep breath causes pain through the liver.
  Bryonia 6c, every 3–4 hours.
- Jaundice caused by haemolytic anemia.
  Crotalus 6c, every 3–4 hours.

Lumbago

Lumbago is pain in the lower part of the back that is commonly caused by injury, arthritis or overstrain of the back muscles. The muscles may be strained or torn, and go into spasm, or ligaments between the vertebrae may be torn. There is often pressure upon the nerves. The pain may be severe and immobilising, and may come on suddenly, making movement difficult. Heat and gentle massage often give benefit. Osteopathic or chiropractic treatment is important: the following remedies will give symptomatic relief.

TREATMENT

- Early stage of lumbago, with inflammation and pain.
  Ferrum phos 6x, a tissue salt, every 3–4 hours.
- Sharp pain, coming on suddenly, made worse by exposure to dry, cold winds.
  Aconite 6c, every 30 minutes for a few doses.
- Pain immediately after injury or overstrain, feels bruised and stiff.
  Arnica 6c, every 3–4 hours.
- Lower back feels stiff and bruised, worse from damp, cold weather, while at rest and in bed. Feels as if must move often to get more comfortable, but only relieves for a while.
  Rhus tox 6c, every 3–4 hours.
- Lumbago from an over-acid condition of the tissue, with sour perspiration.
  Nat phos 6x, a tissue salt, every 3–4 hours.

- Lumbago relieved by lying on something hard, with pain as if bruised from prolonged stooping. Sensation of coldness up and down the spine.
  Nat mur 6x, a tissue salt, every 3–4 hours.
- Pain made worse by the slightest movement, better from pressure and lying on the affected part.
  Bryonia 6c, every 3–4 hours.
- Stiffness and pain worse on the approach of storms.
  Rhododendron 6c, every 3–4 hours.
- Lumbago following exposure to cold and damp, worse by moving or stooping.
  Dulcamara 6c, every 3–4 hours.
- Backache and stiffness from a slight draught, worse in the morning.
  Calc phos 6x, a tissue salt, every 3–4 hours.
- Lumbago following a strain.
  Calc fluor 6x, a tissue salt, every 3–4 hours.

Meningitis

Meningitis is a viral or bacterial infection of the delicate membranes of the brain. Symptoms are fever, nausea and vomiting, a stiff neck, a severe headache made worse by bending forward, intolerance of light and abnormal sleepiness and drowsiness. This disorder is potentially more serious in infants and toddlers than in older children and adults, as there is a risk of brain damage. The symptoms in infants can be a little different, and include an unusually high-pitched cry, coupled with vomiting and intolerance of light. Recovery from viral meningitis takes 2–3 weeks, and is usually complete, but the consequences of the bacterial form can be more serious, and include loss of hearing, brain damage and even death.

*If meningitis is suspected, the following remedies can be tried while allopathic advice is being **urgently sought**.*

TREATMENT

- After head injury.
  Arnica 6c, every 30 minutes.
- With restlessness, great fear, dry skin and intense thirst.
  Aconite 6c, every 30 minutes.
- Hot, delirious, with staring eyes.
  Belladonna 6c, every 30 minutes.
- Severe headache, made worse by the slightest eye movement, wants to lie still and quiet.
  Bryonia 6c, every 30 minutes.
- Infant irritable and oversensitive, with sudden piercing screams.
  Apis 6c, every 30 minutes.

Mouth Ulcers

Mouth ulcers can be very painful and they can have an obscure cause. They can come in crops or singly, can be infrequent or recurrent. They may accompany thrush, and may become infected.

- Ulcers with a gray base on the inside of the cheeks or on the tongue, starting as small vesicles, and made painful by acid or salty foods.
Borax 6c, *every 3–4 hours.*
- Ulcers, shallow and burning, with foul breath, increased salivation and thirst. Tongue may be thick and coated.
Mercurius 6c, *every 3–4 hours.*
- Mouth ulcers on the tongue and the inside of the cheeks. Lips and mouth are either excessively dry, or there may be copious salivation. Often there are cold sores on the lips.
Nat mur 6x, *a tissue salt, every 3–4 hours.*
- Ulcers with white membrane and often a thick, white discharge. The tongue is coated white.
Kali mur 6x, *a tissue salt, every 3–4 hours.*
- Ulcers ashy-gray, especially from nervous stress.
Kali phos 6x, *a tissue salt, every 3–4 hours.*
- Ulcers with a yellowish membrane, anywhere in the mouth.
Kali bich 6c, *every 3–4 hours.*
- Ulcers with irregular edges, bleeding easily with a pricking, stinging pain.
Nit ac 6c, *every 3–4 hours.*
- Ulcers secreting a thick, yellowish mucus, especially on the inside of the lower lip.
Hydrastis 6c, *every 3–4 hours.*
- Gums sore, with blisters becoming ulcers. Ulcerated corners of the mouth and cold sores on lips.
Rhus tox 6c, *every 3–4 hours.*
- Whitish or yellowish ulcerations that bleed easily, with foul breath and profuse salivation.
Sulph ac 6c, *every 3–4 hours.*

Neuralgia and Nerve Pain

Neuralgia is a severe, sharp pain along the course of a nerve. It is due to a painful inflammation of nerve fibres, and is usually worse from cold or draughts. It occurs anywhere in the body, but most notably in the trigeminal nerve of the face. Osteopathic or chiropractic treatment should always be considered.

- For intense, darting, excruciating or spasmodic pain, relieved by heat and pressure, and aggravated by cold.
  Mag phos 6x, a tissue salt, every 3–4 hours.
- Neuralgic pain coming on suddenly, after sudden exposure to cold or cold, dry winds.
  Aconite 6c, every 30 minutes for a few doses.
- Attack brought on by dry cold. Person feels chilly, exhausted and restless, with burning pains relieved by heat.
  Arsenicum alb 6c, every 3–4 hours.
- Neuralgic pain violent and cutting, especially in the face, brought on by cold or damp and relieved by heat.
  Colocynthis 6c, every 3–4 hours.
- Paralysing pain in sensitive persons, better by gentle motion and when mind is occupied. Often with insomnia, irritability, exhaustion and oversensitivity.
  Kali phos 6x, a tissue salt, every 3–4 hours.
- Severe neuralgic pain, but intermittent, with excessive flow of saliva.
  Nat mur 6x, a tissue salt, every 3–4 hours.
- Severe, throbbing neuralgic pain, like a nail being driven in over the eye, with burning heat and a flushed face.
  Ferrum phos 6x, a tissue salt, every 3–4 hours.
- Pains coming on at night, with a sensation of numb crawling or coldness, especially in anemic persons.
  Calc phos 6x, a tissue salt, every 3–4 hours.
- Neuralgia brought on by damp weather or by living in a damp house.
  Nat sulph 6x, a tissue salt, every 3–4 hours.
- Neuralgia affecting the rib cage, or above the right eye.
  Ranunculus 6c, every 3–4 hours.
- Neuralgia above the left eye, made worse by movement.
  Spigelia 6c, every 3–4 hours.

Perspiration, Offensive

Sweating is an important mechanism for the body to reduce body heat and eliminate wastes. Homeopathically speaking, it is not healthy to suppress perspiration with anti-perspirants. However, offensive-smelling sweat may indicate a constitutional imbalance that should be treated.

- Overweight, clammy persons, easily fearful, with sour sweat, especially round the head at night.
  Calc carb 6c, every 3–4 hours.
- Thin, chilly persons, with profuse offensive sweat on the feet, must change socks often.
  Silicea 6x, a tissue salt, every 3–4 hours.
- Perspiration greasy, pungent and unpleasant; it is worse at night and by both heat and cold.
  Mercurius 6c, every 3–4 hours.

- Sweating worse about the head, sour-smelling and profuse, better by cold weather and by walking.
  Fluoric ac 6c, every 3–4 hours.
- Excessive perspiration with sour, acidic smell and tongue coated creamy at the back.
  Nat phos 6x, a tissue salt, every 3–4 hours.
- Sweats are easy, profuse and offensive, in overweight persons with dry, harsh skin and poor circulation.
  Graphites 6c, every 3–4 hours.

Psoriasis

Psoriasis is a complex and chronic inflammatory disease of the skin, with unsightly patches of pink, raised, flaking skin on the knees, elbows, lower back, and the scalp behind the ears. In a few cases, the joints of the hands, fingers, knees and ankles may become inflamed and swollen. Orthodox treatments manage but do not cure the condition and include steroid and coal tar ointments, cytotoxic ointments that slow down cell division, vitamin A and D derivatives that can be highly toxic, and ultraviolet therapy. The remedies given below have a long history of success, but there are many remedies that may suit, and for such a chronic condition a constitutional treatment from a homeopath is recommended. If any remedy causes aggravation, stop giving it immediately and wait for the aggravation to die down and improvement to set in. Give another dose only when improvement stops.

- Skin is thick and dry, especially at the fingertips, bends of the limbs, the orifices, behind the ears and on the face and scalp. The skin may crack, itch and bleed, and ooze a honey-coloured exudate. The itch is worse for warmth, the heat of the bed and washing, and is better by cold.
  Graphites 6c, morning and evening.
- Skin is hot, dry, red, scaly and itchy, worse from heat and washing, and worse at night from the heat of the bed. May put feet out of bed at night to cool.
  Sulphur 6c, morning and evening.

- Skin is dry and scaly, with burning sensation relieved by heat, often worse around midnight.
  Arsenicum 6c, morning and evening.
- Psoriasis better during the summer, and notably worse during winter and from cold.
  Petroleum 6c, morning and evening.
- Skin itchy and unhealthy, may crack, peel and bleed, and have a musty, mousy odor. It is always worse from heat, at night, washing, contact with wool, and the heat of the bed.
  Psorinum 30c, one dose per week.

Rheumatism

Rheumatism is a general term for pain and stiffness of the muscles and joints. The pains are usually worse in cold, damp weather, and are better by warmth and massage. Orthodox treatment is with anti-inflammatory drugs and pain killers. Homeopathic treatment is constitutional, but the following remedies can be used first, and will give relief if well suited.

TREATMENT

Vegetarian diet suits best, because of its alkaline-forming qualities. For those unable or unwilling to adopt such a diet, avoid wheat, rye, oats, barley, meat, dairy products, potatoes, tomatoes, capsicum and eggplant as much as possible. Restrict tea, coffee, alcohol and spices.

- In the first stages, with heat, pain and redness. Pains are increased by movement.
  Ferrum phos 6x, a tissue salt, every 3–4 hours.
- Second stage of rheumatism or fibrositis, when swelling has resulted, and movement increases the pains. Thick white or grayish coating on the tongue.
  Kali mur 6x, a tissue salt, every 3–4 hours.
- Pain and stiffness, causing great restlessness, often brought on by cold and damp, and improved by heat. Pains are worse on initial movement, especially in the morning, but better on continued movement, after limbering up.
  Rhus tox 6c, every 3–4 hours.
- Rheumatism from over-acid conditions of the tissue, with sour-smelling sweat and an acid taste in the mouth. Tongue is coated creamy-yellow at the base.
  Nat phos 6x, a tissue salt, every 3–4 hours.
- Stabbing pain better when absolutely still, worse on movement and in dry, cold weather, and relieved by pressure and lying on the affected part.
  Bryonia 6c, every 3–4 hours.
- Pain made worse by heat and warm rooms, flitting from one part of the body to another.
  Pulsatilla 6c, every 3–4 hours.

- Rheumatism that is worse by humidity and at every change of weather and better by dry, settled weather. The tongue is clear, or has a gray–green coating at the base.
  Nat sulph 6x, a tissue salt, every 3–4 hours.
- Rheumatism with stiffness and numbness, that is worse at night, from heat or cold, dampness, and at every change of weather.
  Calc phos 6x, a tissue salt, every 3–4 hours.
- Pain mainly in the jaw and neck, with muscle spasm, better in warm, damp or humid weather.
  Causticum 6c, every 3–4 hours.
- Pain and stiffness worse in cold, damp weather, especially after becoming overheated.
  Dulcamara 6c, every 3–4 hours.
- Enlargement of the joints from rheumatism.
  Calc fluor 6x, a tissue salt, every 3–4 hours.
- Acute, sharp, spasmodic pains in rheumatism, relieved by pressure, massage or warmth.
  Mag phos 6x, a tissue salt, every 3–4 hours.
- Joints feel cold and numb, with pain and stiffness increasing when the weather changes.
  Calc phos 6x, a tissue salt, every 3–4 hours.

- Stiff, bruised pains after injury, no matter how long ago.
  Arnica 6c, every 3–4 hours.
- Bruised, sore, aching stiffness, feels that he or she must move, but no better by it.
  Phytolacca 6c, every 3–4 hours.
- Pain worse when at rest and better by motion, and particularly aggravated by the approach of stormy weather.
  Rhododendron 6c, every 3–4 hours.

- Limbs stiff and painful after taking cold, or when the weather changes from warm to cold, somewhat better by movement.
  Dulcamara 6c, every 3–4 hours.
- Aches and pains worse at night, with greasy, offensive sweat and foul taste in the mouth in the morning.
  Mercurius 6c, every 3–4 hours.
- Pain in the joints, especially the larger ones, where the tendons meet the bone, better by warmth.
  Ruta grav 6c, every 3–4 hours.

Sciatica

Sciatica is pain in the sciatic nerve, which supplies the legs. It is caused by nerve inflammation or injury, usually because of pressure from a misaligned spine, a damaged or prolapsed disc, or from osteoarthritis. It shows as a sharp, shooting pain into the buttock and leg, especially when bending, sneezing or coughing. Orthodox treatment includes pain killers, muscle relaxants, steroid injections and physiotherapy. Osteopathy, chiropractic and acupuncture usually offer more lasting benefit. The following remedies can be taken for relief in acute cases.

TREATMENT

- Pain coming on quickly, especially after exposure to cold or dry cold wind, with anxiety and restlessness.
  Aconite 6c, every 1–2 hours.

- For general pain and inflammation.
  Ferrum phos 6x, a tissue salt, every 3–4 hours.

- Cramping, lightning-like pains, especially in the right leg, worse by coughing and better by heat.
  Mag phos 6x, a tissue salt, every 3–4 hours.
- Sciatic pain in the elderly, worse at night around midnight causing restlessness, and better by warmth.
  Arsenicum 6c, every 3–4 hours.
- Pain shoots down the right leg, with numbness and weakness, worse in cold or damp weather.
  Colocynthis 6c, every 3–4 hours.
- Pain worse when sitting. Difficulty straightening the affected leg because the muscle and tendon have contracted; better by walking and rest.
  Ammonium mur 6c, every 3–4 hours.
- Pain with cramping and pronounced numbness in the affected leg, the numbness alternating with the pain. Better by rest and worse by movement.
  Gnaphalium 6c, every 3–4 hours.
- Shifting, shooting pains, returning regularly, especially in the left leg, with increasing stiffness and difficulty in walking, and worse by both heat and cold.
  Carbon sulph 6c, every 3–4 hours.
- Burning pains shooting into the knee and foot, can come any time but especially around 3 a.m., causing cries of pain.
  Kali carb 6c, every 3–4 hours.
- Cramping, tearing pain, better by heat and movement, worse from cold, damp, and by rest in bed, driving to move restlessly, which improves for a while.
  Rhus tox 6c, every 3–4 hours.
- Pain in the right leg, aggravated by pressure and lying on the right side, and often coming on 4–8 p.m.
  Lycopodium 6c, every 3–4 hours.
- Pain with exhaustion; person is irritable, sleepless and sensitive to every stimulus.
  Kali phos 6x, a tissue salt, every 3–4 hours.

Shingles

Shingles is a rash caused by the chickenpox virus, and can be very painful. The rash begins as a burning, stinging pain that may be anywhere, and soon resolves into patches of vesicles, which burst and form scabs. The vesicles follow the course of a nerve, causing inflammation of the skin, with such pain as to make movement, the touch of clothes and pressure on the affected part to be unbearable. Sleep may be impossible, and the patient may be feverish, with aches, pains and malaise. The duration of the disease is normally 14–20 days, or even longer, but this can be dramatically shortened using the appropriate remedy, and the neuralgia that often follows can be avoided.

TREATMENT

■ To be prescribed in the early stages, as soon as the disorder initiates, to shorten the course.
Staphylococcinum 30c, one dose every 3 hours for 2 days.

For established cases

■ Small vesicles the size of pinheads, containing a clear liquid, with itching and burning, not helped by scratching. Patient is restless, and changes position often. The eruption is eased by heat and hot applications.
Rhus tox 6c, every 3–4 hours.

■ Small vesicles like those of Rhus tox symptom picture, but much more numerous and itchier, and more likely to ulcerate.
Rhus ven 6c, every 3–4 hours.

■ Vesicles itch and burn intensely, relieved by heat, often worse after midnight. Patient is restless and anxious, then often exhausted.
Arsenicum 6c, every 3–4 hours.

■ Vesicles are large and sometimes confluent, with a prickly, burning, stinging sensation, helped by cold applications. Usually there is no thirst.
Apis 6c, every 3–4 hours.

■ Itching, burning vesicles containing white or yellow liquid, forming thick crusts covering an underlying ulcer with white or yellowish pus. The pain is worse by movement and the heat of the bed, but better from warmth.
Mezereum 6c, every 3–4 hours.

■ Burning and itching in vesicles, often with shocks and stabs of pain from touch or movement. The blisters may be bluish, with bloodstained fluid.
Ranunculus bulb 6c, every 3–4 hours.

■ Vesicles on the face, with eye pain and the sensation that the eyeball will burst.
Prunus spinosa 6c, every 3–4 hours.

■ Large blisters itching and burning, may be bloody, better by cool air and cold compresses.
Cantharis 6c, every 3–4 hours.

- Itching, painful blisters that, once healed, cover over with a layer of skin on which a new vesicle forms.
Anagallis arvensis 6c, every 3–4 hours.

- As a preventative, for family and friends.
Varicella 30c or *Herpes zoster nosode 30c*, 1 dose per day for 7 days.

Sinusitis

Sinusitis is a complication of acute colds or influenza. Usually there is facial pain, a persistent discharge from the front and back of the nose, and this is often accompanied by nasal blockage. Headache is frequently present and may be severe. Sinus infections can easily become chronic. Acute sinusitis responds well to homeopathic treatment, but chronic sinusitis is difficult because it is often accompanied by long-standing and often irreversible changes to the structure of the sinuses.

TREATMENT

Check for allergic foods in the diet, particularly grains and dairy products, and avoid if possible.

- First stage, with fever, inflammation and pain in the sinuses. The face may be flushed, and the pulse rapid.
Ferrum phos 6x, a tissue salt, every 3–4 hours.

- In the early stages, with blocked nose, loss of smell, sneezing, watery discharge and head pain like thousands of tiny hammers, worse in cold air.
Nat mur 6x, a tissue salt, every 3–4 hours.

- Dull, stuffy pain in the sinuses, a thick, white, mucous discharge and a white-coated tongue.
Kali mur 6x, a tissue salt, every 3–4 hours.

- Pains in sinus with sneezing and watery nasal discharge, abundant and burning. Nose red, swollen, with a sensation of constriction at its root, often with stabbing pains. Pain worse by pressure, heat and warm rooms, better in open air.
Kali iodatum 6c, every 3–4 hours.

■ Frontal headache, with pain at the root of the nose, as if blocked. Constant need to blow nose, but little result. Often a dry, irritating, continuous cough, especially at night.
Sticta pul 6c, every 3–4 hours.

■ Yellow, slimy discharge, worse in warm rooms and at night, and better in the open air.
Kali sulph 6x, a tissue salt, every 3–4 hours.

■ The nose is blocked in the cold open air. Chilly and irritable from drafts and better in warm humid weather. Later a thick, offensive discharge appears, smelling like old cheese.
Hepar sulph 6c, every 3–4 hours.

■ Pain above the eyes with nose stuffed up indoors, flowing more freely out of doors. Discharge is changeable, comes and goes, but usually yellow or yellow–green.
Pulsatilla 6c, every 3–4 hours.

■ Pain and pressure outward along the brow, often encircling the eyes, or pain on the upper part of the nose, as if wearing tight spectacles. Radiating pain from the eyes to the sides of the face, with marked redness of the eye. Stringy mucus from back of the nose dropping into throat, must hawk to clear. The pain is better in the open air, and worse at night and from the least touch.
Cinnabaris 6c, every 3–4 hours.

■ Discharge of thick, sticky, yellow or greenish–yellow mucus, may be irritating or bloody, often dripping into the throat. The discharge may form strings or crusts. Pain and pressure at the root of the nose, and often a violent cough. Better by heat and movement and worse from cold, damp and fresh air.
Kali bich 6c, every 3–4 hours.

■ Thick, tenacious, yellow, ropy mucus, raw and irritating, with a yellow, slimy tongue. The throat is red and congested, with streaks of mucus running down from the back of the nose, worse from cold and in the open air.
Hydrastis 6c, every 3–4 hours.

■ Burning pains in the bones of the nose and face, with sneezing, and a yellow discharge, sometimes streaked with blood. Worse at night and the warmth of the bed, and from cold, damp weather.
Mezereum 6c, every 3–4 hours.

■ Sinusitis with foul discharges, fever and agitation, worse from cold and damp, better from heat and pressure. Pyrogen acts similarly to an antibiotic, and can stop the progression towards infection.
Pyrogen 6c, every 3–4 hours.

- Sinusitis often beginning with a headache, which is relieved when discharge appears and returns when discharge is blocked. Worse at night and from sun's heat.
  Lachesis 6c, every 3–4 hours.

- Chronic sinusitis with thick, offensive, acrid discharges, tip of the nose itchy, and ulceration of the nasal mucous membrane.
  Silicea 6x, a tissue salt, every 3–4 hours.

Skin Problems

The skin accounts for about 16 per cent of the total body weight; it is the largest organ of the body. Apart from contact dermatitis, most skin conditions arise from internal problems and general imbalance; it is these problems that must be treated. Diet is often a factor. Even so, in homeopathic medicine some good skin remedies can be prescribed just on the obvious and visible symptoms. In using the following remedies, remember that the treatment of many skin conditions often takes months. Delay giving further doses if the skin gets worse, and wait for improvement to follow. Give further single doses only when the improvement stops, using a higher potency. If there are complications, see a homeopath.

TREATMENT

- Skin and hair dry. Skin flakes easily, hair falls out.
  Nat mur 6x, a tissue salt, every 3–4 hours.

- Thin and softened nails, weak hair, and susceptibility to cold.
  Silicea 6x, a tissue salt, every 3–4 hours.

- Cracked skin, looks rough and red, especially at the corners of the mouth.
  Petroleum 6c, every 3–4 hours.

- Chapping and cracks of the skin, even the palms of the hands. Fissures around the nails, mouth and anus. The skin may become hard, tough. Brittle fingernails.
  Calc fluor 6x, a tissue salt, every 3–4 hours.

- Dry, peeling skin, with or without sticky secretions.
  Kali sulph 6x, a tissue salt, every 3–4 hours.

- Cracking in the nostrils, on lips, behind ears, on nipples, or on fingertips.
  Graphites 6c, every 3–4 hours.
- Cracks on fingertips, becoming deeper in cold weather, slow to heal, with sweaty hands and feet.
  Silicea 6x, a tissue salt, every 3–4 hours.
- Eczema and eruptions of the skin with exhausting perspiration, offensive odor and nervous irritability.
  Kali phos 6x, a tissue salt, every 3–4 hours.
- Cracking in the folds of the skin, especially if complicated by fungal infection. Skin is itchy, worse from washing.
  Sulphur 6c, every 3–4 hours.
- Watery blisters, burning and irritating, with thin, transparent, white scales.
  Nat mur 6x, a tissue salt, every 3–4 hours.
- Skin dry, red and itching, worse from heat, hot water and the warmth of the bed.
  Sulphur 6c, every 3–4 hours.
- Skin becomes red and itchy after water is applied, with clear discharges like the white of an egg.
  Calc phos 6x, a tissue salt, every 3–4 hours.
- Eczema in the bends of the joints.
  Nat mur 6x, a tissue salt, every 3–4 hours.
- Dry, dirty-looking skin, often smells musty, with intolerable itching.
  Psorinum 30c, 1 dose per week for several months.
- Eruptions on any part of the body, when the contents are thick and white, and accompanied by a white-coated tongue.
  Kali mur 6x, a tissue salt, every 3–4 hours.
- Eruptions of the skin when the discharges are watery, yellow and foul.
  Kali sulph 6x, a tissue salt, every 3–4 hours.
- Greenish–yellow exudate, with the formation of crusts.
  Kali sulph 6x, a tissue salt, every 3–4 hours.
- Athlete's foot.
  Kali sulph 6x, a tissue salt, every 3–4 hours.
- Skin eruptions when the discharges are creamy, golden–yellow or colored like honey, with sour sweat and a creamy coating at the back of the tongue.
  Nat phos 6x, a tissue salt, every 3–4 hours.

- Thick yellow discharges from wounds that do not heal easily. Pimples and pustules during adolescence.
  Calc sulph 6x, a tissue salt, every 3–4 hours.

- Boils, abscesses and suppurating, festering sores.
  Hepar sulph 6c, every 3–4 hours.
- Boils and ulcers suppurating easily but healing poorly, with sweaty, offensive feet.
  Silicea 6x, a tissue salt, every 3–4 hours.

Sore Throat

Sore throat is a blanket term that covers disorders of several organs. It must always be treated with attention, as it may be the first symptom in the development of other disorders, such as tonsillitis, laryngitis, pharyngitis or diptheria, that carry additional risk of complication. If homeopathic treatment does not improve a sore throat, allopathic advice should always be sought.

TREATMENT

As a general treatment, gargle a mixed tincture of Cinnamon and Sage, 20 drops of each in a half-glass of water. Alternatively gargle water with a few drops of tea tree oil added, but do not swallow.

- The throat is bright red and shiny; the patient is nervous, sensitive and easily flushed but not anxious. Heat, pain and dryness are marked, and there is no exudation.
  Ferrum phos 6x, a tissue salt, every 3–4 hours. The first remedy to try and often the only remedy needed.

- Sore throat, with fever, anxiety and thirst, painful on speaking or swallowing, with a dry, tingling, burning sensation. Often following exposure to cold, dry wind.
  Aconite 6c, every 1–2 hours.
- Throat red and shiny, face red, pupils enlarged, skin hot and dry. Restlessness. Swallowing is painful, pain may spread to ears.
  Belladonna 6c, every 3–4 hours.

- Sore and swollen throat with high fever and stinging, burning pain, or sometimes no pain at all; but always worse from touch. Tissues have a swollen, glazed, purple–red appearance. Cold drinks and sucking ice always relieve, heat in any form aggravates. Right side is often worse.
  Apis 6c, every 2–3 hours.

- Throat sore, very sensitive to touch and cold air, worse at night. Sensation of a crumb or fishbone in the throat, with pain through to the ears on swallowing.
  Hepar sulph 6c, every 2–3 hours.

- Throat is red, raw, burning and smarting, worse at night and on waking. Tongue coated yellow, breath foul. Thirsty, even though mouth is moist. May bring up yellow mucus, tinged with blood.
  Mercurius 6c, every 3–4 hours.

- Like symptom picture for Mercurius, but worse on the left side.
  Merc bin iod 6c, every 3–4 hours.

- Throat is dry, irritable, pricking and painful; worse from any type of motion—talking, swallowing or turning the head—and better from pressure and stillness. Intense thirst is often, but not always, present.
  Bryonia 6c, every 2–3 hours.

- Like symptom picture for Mercurius, but worse on right.
  Merc iod flav 6c, every 3–4 hours.

- The sore throat develops slowly, person feels tired, heavy, no energy, weak and shaky, hot and cold in turn, with cold shivers up and down the back. Pain in neck and ears made worse by swallowing, patient avoids drinks because swallowing hurts so much. Usually there is no thirst.
  Gelsemium 6c, every 2–3 hours.

- The throat is painfully raw, sore and burning, often from overuse of voice in talking or singing; voice is hoarse or breaks. Although very painful, the throat may be itchy; the patient may often want to grasp or scratch it, even though swallowing is painful. There may be raw cracks in the corners of the mouth, cracks in the centre of the lips and mouth ulcers.
  Arum triphyllum 6c, every 2–3 hours.

- Frothy, transparent mucus covering the tongue, with swollen uvula (the flap of skin at the centre back of the mouth) and a sense of obstruction in the throat. Constant flow of clear saliva.
  Nat mur 6x, a tissue salt, every 3–4 hours.

- Swelling of the throat with a white-coated tongue and difficulty swallowing.
  Kali mur 6x, a tissue salt, every 3–4 hours.
- Acute sore throat coming on after exposure to cold and damp, or after exertion. Throat is raw and burning, saliva thick, voice hoarse. There may be cold sores around the mouth, a red, itchy skin as in nettle rash, a thirst for cold drinks and restlessness.
  Dulcamara 6c, every 2–3 hours.
- Pain and soreness on the right side, with feeling of lump in the throat, coming on slowly. Neck glands swollen, lips dry, thirsty but not hungry.
  Baryta mur 6c, every 2–3 hours.
- The throat is swollen, dark red, burning and constricted; the pains are often worse between swallowing. The ears are very tender, with severe, shooting pains. Typically the patient is red and feverish, but is chilly, feels cold, and is worse from cold and draughts. Water is often craved, but it makes the throat worse and increases the chill.
  Capsicum 6c, every 2–3 hours.
- Ulcerated sore throat, with formation of yellow pits.
  Calc sulph 6x, a tissue salt, every 3–4 hours.
- Plugs or lumps in the throat—often as a result of suppressed emotion, grief, or unrequited love. The pain is worse from liquids than solids, typical of the contradictory nature of the remedy, which suits hypersensitive, emotional types, intolerant of contradiction.
  Ignatia 6c, every 3–4 hours.
- Creamy-yellow mucus on the tonsils and the base of the tongue, with sensation of a lump in the throat. There may be acid stomach or sour risings.
  Nat phos 6x, tissue salt, every 3–4 hours.
- Inflamed throat; tonsils swell and become very red at first, then may change to dark or bluish-red, especially on the right side. Shooting pains running into the ears when swallowing, starting at the root of the tongue.
  Phytolacca 6c, every 2–3 hours.
- Sore throat, extremely sensitive, first on one side then the other, and may alternate for days. Feels dry, scalded, tight and stiff, as if it were closing up. Sensation of a lump in throat, and pain through to ears on swallowing. Worse from cold air, better by either warm or cold drinks.
  Lac caninum 6c, every 3–4 hours.
- Relaxed sore throat, with tickling in the larynx.
  Calc fluor 6x, a tissue salt, every 3–4 hours.

Styes

Styes are an infection of the pores of the skin of the eyelid. They look like a boil, occur at the roots of eyelashes and can be very painful.

TREATMENT

- At the onset of appearance.
  Pulsatilla 6c, every 3–4 hours.
- Styes, from resentment or other suppressed emotion.
  Staphysagria 6c, every 3–4 hours.
- Styes in small crops, extremely sensitive to touch and cold air.
  Hepar sulph 6c, every 3–4 hours.

- Bluish styes in small crops.
  Arnica 6c, every 3–4 hours.
- Styes in those who feel cold easily, may have offensive foot sweats.
  Silicea 6x, a tissue salt, every 3–4 hours.

Synovitis

Synovitis is the inflammation of the membrane lining a joint. There is usually a release of fluid into the joint, causing swelling and pain. It may occur in some rheumatic disorders, and also after injury and strain. Bursitis and housemaid's knee are similar conditions.

TREATMENT

- Pain, inflammation and stiffness.
  Ferrum phos 6x, a tissue salt, every 3–4 hours.
- Joint hot, red and painful, throbbing and swollen worse from the slightest jar.
  Belladonna 6c, every 3–4 hours.
- Pain made worse on any movement. Better from strong bandaging and rest.
  Bryonia 6c, every 3–4 hours.

- Joint stiff and swollen with tearing pains, worse by cold damp weather and better by warmth and gentle exercise.
  Rhus tox 6c, every 3–4 hours.
- Synovitis with pain in the joint, worse on first rising from sitting, at night and also worse from the heat of the bed.
  Sulphur 6c, every 3–4 hours.

- Chronic synovitis, with swelling and difficulty of movement.
  Silicea 6x, a tissue salt, every 3–4 hours.

- For long-standing cases that are slow to respond.
  Calc fluor 6x, a tissue salt, every 3–4 hours.

Tonsillitis

Tonsillitis is an inflammation of the tonsils, and may be either acute or chronic. It occurs mainly during winter, with a sudden onset, pain in swallowing, chilliness and fever. The tonsils become enlarged and often show a white exudation. Tonsillitis may involve the glands of the throat, which also become tender and swollen. Most cases resolve easily, although there is always a risk of complication. If a membrane forms in the throat diptheria is to be feared and allopathic treatment should be sought. In the early stages, gargling water with a few drops of tea tree oil added often helps, but do not swallow.

TREATMENT

- Throat bright red, shiny; patient feverish, nervous, sensitive and easily flushed but not anxious. Inflammation marked, but no exudation.
  Ferrum phos 6x, a tissue salt, every 3–4 hours. The first remedy to try and often the only remedy needed.

- Sore throat with swelling of the tonsils, hoarseness and hacking cough, often from taking cold through exposure to draughts, or while damp. Adult is restless and irritable, child is cross, irritable and wishes to be carried.
  Chamomilla 6c, every 1–3 hours.

- Throat bright red, dry and burns like fire, tonsils swollen with pains shooting into the ears, outside of the throat swollen. Patient flushed and restless.
  Belladonna 6c, every 1–2 hours.

- Sore and swollen throat with high fever and stinging, burning pain—or sometimes no pain at all—but always worse from touch. The tissues have a swollen, glazed, purple–red appearance. There is no thirst, but sucking ice will relieve, while heat in any form aggravates. The right side is often worse.
  Apis 6c, every 2–3 hours.

- Swelling of the tonsils with a white-coated tongue and difficulty swallowing. May be white or grey spots on the tonsils.
  Kali mur 6x, a tissue salt, every 3–4 hours.
- Offensive sore throat. Tonsils generally very swollen, with yellow coating on tongue and burning pain into ears. Foul breath, profuse flow of saliva with marked dryness of throat and intense thirst; often an oily sweat. The throat is worse at night, in the mornings, after sleep.
  Mercurius 6c, every 2–3 hours.
- Like Mercurius symptom picture, but worse on the left side.
  Merc bin iod 6c, every 3–4 hours.
- Like Mercurius symptom picture, but worse on the right side.
  Merc iod flav 6c, every 3–4 hours.
- Frothy, transparent mucus covering the tonsils, with swollen uvula (the flap of skin at the centre back of the mouth) and a sense of obstruction in throat. Constant flow of clear saliva.
  Nat mur 6x, a tissue salt, every 3–4 hours.
- Creamy, yellow mucus on the tonsils and the base of the tongue, with sensation of a lump in the throat. There may be acid stomach or sour risings.
  Nat phos 6x, a tissue salt, every 3–4 hours.
- Tongue and back of the throat

- Inflamed throat; tonsils swell and become very red at first, then may change to dark or bluish red, especially on the right side. Shooting pains running into the ears when swallowing, starting at the root of the tongue. White or gray-white spots appear on tonsils, coalescing to form patches.
  Phytolacca 6c, every 2–3 hours.
- Sore throat, extremely sensitive, first on one side then the other, and may alternate for days. Feels dry, scalded, tight and stiff, as if it were closing up. Sensation of a lump in the throat, and pain through to the ears on swallowing. Worse from cold air, better by either warm or cold drinks.
  Lac caninum 6c, every 3–4 hours.
- Pitted sore throat, white pits full of pus and debris, with extreme sensitivity to pain, cold air and draughts. Violent pricking pains when swallowing, running into the ears or the glands of the throat, and a sensation of a splinter at the back of throat.
  Hepar sulph 6c, every 2–3 hours.
- Tonsils and throat are bright red and ulcerated, with a sensation of constriction. Swallowing is difficult, and there is fear of any contact or pressure.
  Lachesis 6c, every 3–4 hours.
- Repeated tonsillitis in those with

yellowish and coated. The tonsils may be suppurating or abscessed; there is a craving for fresh air.
Calc sulph 6x, a tissue salt, every 3–4 hours.

■ Repeated tonsillitis in children or adults with chronically enlarged tonsils and lymphatic glands.
Baryta carb 6c, every 3–4 hours.

chronically enlarged tonsils, and who suffer periodic fevers, colds and influenza.
Tuberculinum 30c, 1 dose per month.

Toothache

Decayed teeth should always receive dental care, especially if infection is suspected. If there is throbbing, swelling of the gum or face, and a rise in temperature, an infection or abscess may be developing.

TREATMENT

■ As a local application on swelling or painful area.
Hypericum tincture, or oil of cloves.

■ To relieve the anxiety before visiting dentist.
Aconite 6c, every 30 minutes.

■ Before and after visit to dentist, to relieve the pain of extraction. Arnica is a wonderful remedy.
Arnica 200c, 1 dose before the extraction and 1 dose after.

■ Enamel of the teeth rough and deficient, causing rapid decay. Teeth loose in their sockets.
Calc fluor 6x, a tissue salt, every 3–4 hours, for 1 month.

■ Inflamed toothache, with redness and swelling.
Ferrum phos 6x, a tissue salt, every 3–4 hours.

■ Stabbing pain with restlessness, especially after ice cream, cold foods or cold wind.
Aconite 6c, every 1–2 hours.

■ Restless and flushed, with congested face and throbbing pain.
Belladonna 6c, every 2–3 hours.

■ Irritable, restless, thirsty and hot. Pain is worse at night and from warm food or drink.
Chamomilla 6c, every 2–3 hours.

- Toothache with salivation, teeth very sensitive to touch, feel longer than normal.
  Plantago 6c, every 3–4 hours.
- Pain with foul mouth, stabbing pain to the ear. Increased thirst and saliva. Worse from hot and cold, better from rubbing the cheek.
  Mercurius 6c, every 3–4 hours.
- Teeth sensitive to touch and cold, with severe, shooting pains.
  Mag phos 6x, a tissue salt, every 3–4 hours.
- Teeth very sensitive to touch or cold, with drawing and tearing pain, irritability and resentment. Cheek may be swollen and red.
  Staphysagria 6c, every 3–4 hours.
- Severe pain in decayed or filled teeth, from oversensitivity of the nerve.
  Kali phos 6x, a tissue salt, every 3–4 hours.
- Intolerable pain, forcing patient to pace restlessly.
  Chamomilla 6c, every 3–4 hours.
- Toothache relieved by holding cold water in the mouth.
  Bryonia 6c, every 3–4 hours.
- Bad teeth, bad breath and bitter taste.
  Kreosote 6c, every 3–4 hours.
- Local pain, with stinging and throbbing, often with swelling of the gum.
  Apis 6c, every 3–4 hours.
- Gum is hot, shining and swollen, but pus or abscess is not obvious.
  Belladonna 6c, every 2–3 hours.
- For swelling with suspected abscess, to speed up ripening.
  Hepar sulph 6c, every 3–4 hours.
- Abscess discharging pus, with foul taste and feverish state.
  Pyrogen 6c, every 3–4 hours.

Travel Sickness

Travel sickness includes seasickness and airsickness, and is a distressing condition caused by the rhythmic or irregular movements associated with travelling. Symptoms range from simple nausea or headache to vomiting and collapse. Influences likely to improve the condition are fresh air, and freedom from smells of petroleum, cooking and tobacco. A tea made from fresh ginger root often relieves.

TREATMENT

■ Persistent nausea, with accumulation of water in the mouth. Worse from passive motion, from light, noise or attempting to sit up. Better from closing the eyes, and from eating small amounts of food.
Petroleum 6c, every 1–2 hours.

■ Nausea and giddiness, with death-like pallor, icy coldness and sweat; may faint. Violent vomiting with cold sweat. Worse by least motion and tobacco smoke; better from cold, and in fresh cold air.
Tabacum 6c, every 1–2 hours.

■ Nausea and vomiting from travel motion, or even from looking at a boat in motion; wants to lie down and be still, better by fixing eyes on the horizon. Sick headache, with inclination to vomit, worse from sight or smell of food. Great weakness, hollow, "gone" feeling. Better from warmth.
Cocculus 6c, every 1–2 hours.

■ Nausea worse from any downward motion, such as in aircraft and lifts.
Borax 6c, every 1–2 hours.

Varicose Veins

Varicose veins are veins that have become stretched and dilated, and are especially found on the inner side of the leg. When they occur in the lower end of the bowel they are known as hemorrhoids. A tendency to varicose veins is often hereditary, and jobs that require long standing with little opportunity to move about can also lead to them. Varicose veins can also appear during pregnancy, although they often disappear after the child is born.

TREATMENT

Elevate the legs as often as possible, and apply tincture of **Hamamelis** externally as a compress. If available, take the minerals calcium fluoride and silica.

- Inflammation of the veins, sore and throbbing, with red streaks following the course of the vein, better by walking slowly.
  Ferrum phos 6x, a tissue salt, every 3–4 hours.
- Varicose veins with bluish discoloration of the tissue.
  Calc fluor 6x, a tissue salt, every 3–4 hours.
- Varicose veins with sore, bruised feeling in the legs.
  Hamamelis 6c, every 3–4 hours.
- Varicose veins, aching, swollen and purple, often with a sore, lame back.
  Aesculus 6c, every 3–4 hours.
- Aching, throbbing veins, with shooting pains along the leg.
  Belladonna 6c, every 3–4 hours.
- Varicose veins during pregnancy, with sore, bruised feeling in the legs, worse from warmth and allowing the legs to hang down.
  Pulsatilla 6c, every 3–4 hours.
- Varicose veins with severe, spasmodic, cramping pains.
  Mag phos 6x, a tissue salt, every 3–4 hours.
- Varicose veins, worse when the legs are allowed to hang down, with pain as if they would burst.
  Vipera 6c, every 3–4 hours.

Vertigo

Vertigo, otherwise known as giddiness, is the sensation of moving around in space, or of having objects moving about the person. It is due to a disturbance of the balancing apparatus in the ear, and may be caused by middle-ear disease, spinal misalignment, infectious disease, low blood pressure, or toxic conditions from smoking, excess alcohol or environmental pollutants. It is a side effect of many drugs.

TREATMENT

Check for environmental causes, and seek chiropractic or osteopathic advice.
- Giddiness from a rush of blood to the head, with flushing or throbbing pain.
  Ferrum phos 6x, a tissue salt, every 3–4 hours.
- Vertigo worse when rising suddenly, particularly after a blow or injury to the head.
  Arnica 6c, every 3–4 hours.

- Vertigo worse from rising or looking upwards, from nervous causes.
  Kali phos 6x, a tissue salt, every 3–4 hours.
- Vertigo worse when closing the eyes, when sitting or lying down, and worse from loud noise.
  Theridion 6c, every 3–4 hours.
- Vertigo worse when lying down or turning over in bed.
  Conium 6c, every 3–4 hours.
- Vertigo worse when sitting, with nausea and a tendency to vomit or faint.
  Cocculus 6c, every 3–4 hours.
- Vertigo from heights or from looking up at tall buildings.
  Arg nit 6c, every 3–4 hours.
- Vertigo with great fear of downward motion.
  Borax 6c, every 3–4 hours.
- Vertigo with trembling and weakness, as if the muscles refuse to obey the will.
  Gelsemium 6c, every 3–4 hours.
- Vertigo worse when trying to walk, turn or read, can come on suddenly.
  Kali carb 6c, every 3–4 hours.
- Vertigo with bitter taste in mouth and tendency to fall to right side, from upset stomach.
  Nat sulph 6x, a tissue salt, every 3–4 hours.
- Vertigo from optical disorders, with black spots before the eyes.
  Mag phos 6x, a tissue salt, every 3–4 hours.
- Dizziness worse in cold weather and when lying on the left side.
  Silicea 6c, every 3–4 hours.

Vomiting

Vomiting can be merely one symptom in a much larger picture, such as in pregnancy or during influenza, and in such cases the appropriate section should also be checked for additional remedies. Generally vomiting is no great cause for concern unless it is persistent, especially in infants and young children. In these cases, care should be taken to replace lost fluids, and allopathic advice should be sought in intractable cases.

- Nausea **not relieved by vomiting**—nothing relieves. With nausea is profuse saliva; vomiting can be food, bile, blood, mucus. May be diarrhea. Ipecac leads all nausea remedies.
Ipecac 6c, every 3–4 hours.

- Intense but not persistent nausea, with thirst for cold water, little and often, and relief after vomiting. General coldness, drowsiness, prostration and sweat.
Ant tart 6c, every 3–4 hours.

- Burning of whole digestive tract—tongue, throat, esophagus, stomach, even to anus; with vomiting, sour, sweetish or bitter, burning the throat. Profuse saliva and ropy mucus, which hangs in strings.
Iris vers 6c, every 3–4 hours.

- Nausea and vomiting, relieved by very hot water, and particularly if there is a pain under the right shoulder blade. May have yellow tint to skin, tongue and eyes.
Chelidonium 6c, every 3–4 hours.

- Vomiting in pregnancy, with "all gone" feeling, especially if the thought or smell of food sickens.
Sepia 6c, every 3–4 hours.

- Persistent nausea, with accumulation of water in the mouth. Worse from passive motion, light, noise or trying to sit up. Petroleum is a good remedy in travel sickness.
Petroleum 6c, every 3–4 hours.

- Nausea and giddiness, with death-like pallor, icy coldness and sweat. Seasickness, worse by least motion, better on deck in fresh, cold air. Violent vomiting with cold sweat, on moving, during pregnancy.
Tabacum 6c, every 3–4 hours.

- Nausea, vomiting, with sweat, prostration, shortness of breath. Profuse watery saliva. Worse: tobacco, slightest motion.
Lobelia 6c, every 3–4 hours.

- Nausea and vomiting from riding in a plane, car or boat, or even looking at a boat in motion. Sick headache from travelling, with inclination to vomit. Great weakness, hollow "gone" feeling. Cocculus is useful for any kind of travel sickness.
Cocculus 6c, every 3–4 hours.

- Exhaustion after loss of fluids from persistent vomiting.
China 6c, every 3–4 hours.

Warts

Warts are small, horny outgrowths of skin, commonly occurring on the hands, but can be anywhere. Treatment should continue for several weeks, then wait.

TREATMENT

Locally, apply tincture of *Thuja* twice a day.

- Warts on the palms of the hands and soles of the feet, or warts that are hard and corny. Both often occur in clusters.
  Ant crud 6c, every 3–4 hours.
- Flat, transparent warts, often on the backs of the hands, and more visible in reflected light than in direct light.
  Dulcamara 6c, every 3–4 hours.
- Warts on the fingertips, under the nails, on the eyelids or on the end of the nose.
  Causticum 6c, every 3–4 hours.
- Soft, fleshy, cauliflower-like warts, that ooze and bleed easily, often on the back of the head.
  Thuja 6c, every 3–4 hours.
- Numerous, small, horny warts that itch, sting, weep and bleed, in chilly persons, sweating easily and always better by warmth.
  Calc carb 6c, every 3–4 hours.
- Warts with a yellow tinge, often with cracking of the skin elsewhere.
  Nit ac 6c, every 3–4 hours.
- Warts that are flat, hollowed out, or raised on tiny stalks.
  Causticum 6c, every 3–4 hours.
- Cauliflower-like warts, often on the upper lip, that itch and sting, ooze and bleed, or become large and jagged.
  Nit ac 6c, every 3–4 hours.
- Warts around the fingernails.
  Graphites 6c, every 3–4 hours.
- Large, dark warts, very fleshy, as if full of water.
  Dulcamara 6c, every 3–4 hours.
- Weeping, ulcerated warts on the tips of the toes.
  Nat carb 6c, every 3–4 hours.
- Large, black warts with hairs in them.
  Sepia 6c, every 3–4 hours.
- Warts around the anus or the genitals, often with numbness and burning.
  Sabina 6c, every 3–4 hours.
- Warts on the foreskin, often bleeding.
  Cinnabar 6c, every 3–4 hours.

5
The Treatment
of Infants

The problems of infants and children represent a special area of medicine. For the most part, the illnesses are mild and rarely life-threatening, while drug treatment is often inappropriate due to problems of toxicity.

It is in this area that homeopathic medicine has much to offer, but remember that babies can become seriously ill much more quickly than adults and children. If well-indicated remedies fail to give improvement, professional advice should always be sought.

The problems of infants usually revolve around feeding disorders and skin rashes. Usually the problem is that the baby cannot tolerate milk, vomits it, has wind or colic, or has diarrhea. Skin disorders include cradle cap, nappy rash and thrush. There also may be irritability, sleeplessness, and crying without apparent cause.

For more general disorders that are as applicable to adults as infants, consult Chapter 3, "Common Problems."

Colic

Intestinal colic is an attack of abdominal pain caused by contractions of the intestines, most common during the first three months of life. Pulling up of the arms and legs, restlessness, crying loudly and turning red in the face are common symptoms, eased by belching and passing gas. In a breast-fed baby, colic can be caused by maternal tension and anxiety, a reaction to dairy products, wheat, beans, cabbage or citrus fruits in the maternal diet, or the baby being held at an extreme angle while feeding, causing air swallowing. In a bottle-fed baby, colic may also be due to air swallowing because the hole in the nipple is too small.

TREATMENT

■ Colic with drawing up of the legs, and relieved by heat and bending double, not relieved by belching. Mag phos is often the only remedy needed.
Mag phos 6x, a tissue salt, every 2–3 hours.

■ Colic with distension and wind, cannot keep still, writhes and twists, with pale face and no thirst. Eased by bending double, firm pressure or a hot water bottle.
Colocynthis 6c, every 2–3 hours.

■ Irritable, restless infant, drawing legs toward abdomen, wanting to be held.
Chamomilla 6c, every 2–3 hours.

■ Distension of abdomen, with green and watery diarrhea.
Chamomilla 6c, every 2–3 hours.

■ Colic, stretches backwards, worse when doubling up and from pressure, with hiccup and sour wind.
Dioscorea 6c, every 2–3 hours.

■ Colic due to poor assimilation of milk or food, if Mag phos fails.
Calc phos 6x, a tissue salt, every 3–4 hours.

■ Colic with sour regurgitations and green, sour-smelling stools.
Nat phos 6x, a tissue salt, every 3–4 hours.

■ Irritable, wants to lie still, and screams at the slightest movement.
Bryonia 6c, every 2–3 hours.

■ Irritable with severe bloating, worse from pressure, often as a result of overfeeding.
Nux vomica 6c, every 2–3 hours.

- Child flushed and restless, with hot and distended abdomen relieved by bending backwards, worse from touch and pressure.
  Belladonna 6c, *every 1–2 hours.*
- Miserable and changeable, may be vomiting milk, wanting to be picked up.
  Pulsatilla 6c, *every 2–3 hours.*

- Colic towards evening, with hardness of abdomen.
  China 6c, *every 2–3 hours.*
- Colic due to irregular contraction of the bile duct, with vomiting of bile, and brownish–green coating on the tongue.
  Nat sulph 6x, *a tissue salt, every 3–4 hours.*

Constipation

Constipation occurs when the bowel is not cleared regularly. A bowel movement 1–3 times a day is considered normal. In infants constipation is not unusual, but should resolve quickly. Commercial laxatives should be avoided: a homemade jelly using agar instead of gelatine, with 25g of agar to half a litre of boiling water, adding half a litre of fruit juice as it cools, is easily taken by a child and helps keep the bowels loose. Sudden cessation of bowel motions, especially in a newborn child, should be viewed with concern, and allopathic advice sought if the condition persists for more than 24 hours.

TREATMENT

- Stool is dry and difficult, child is irritable and thirsty.
  Bryonia 6c, *every 2–3 hours.*
- Straining at stool, but passing only a little at a time. Alternating constipation and diarrhea.
  Nux vomica 6c, *every 2–3 hours.*
- Constipation in chubby babies with sour sweat, especially around the head at night.
  Calc carb 6c, *every 2–3 hours.*

- Even soft stool is passed with difficulty. The child smells sour, despite bathing.
  Hepar sulph 6c, *every 2–3 hours.*
- Constipation of infants, with occasional attacks of diarrhea.
  Nat phos 6x, *a tissue salt, every 3–4 hours.*

Convulsions

Convulsions in infants, toddlers and small children are always alarming, but usually look worse than they are. Not all involutary, convulsive movements are epileptic fits or caused by brain injury or infection: in two-thirds of cases, no cause can be found. These infantile convulsions usually occur during fever or teething, and show as twitching or spasms of limbs or body. The child may become purple during the spasm and hold the breath. **Cooling the child** if there is fever, and giving the appropriate remedy, is usually sufficient. If the fits continue, or the child loses consciousness, allopathic advice should be sought.

TREATMENT

- As an immediate treatment.
  Rub upper lip, below the nose, with tincture of **Camphor**.
- Convulsions during teething, with nightmares and anxiety.
  Aconite 6c, *every 1–2 hours*.
- Convulsions during teething, with heat, flushed face, delirium and restlessness.
  Belladonna 6c, *every 1–2 hours*.
- Convulsions during teething, with restlessness, irritability, and thirst.
  Chamomilla 6c, *every 2–3 hours*.
- Jumps and jerks in sleep, bores fingers into nose and grinds teeth.
  Cina 6c, *every 2–3 hours*.

- With great anger and irritation, and chewing motion of the jaws.
  Nux vomica 6c, *every 2–3 hours*.
- During fever, with jerking of fingers and toes.
  Belladonna 6c, *every 1–2 hours*.
- Convulsion with clammy, sticky hands, exhaustion and sleep. May vomit.
  Aethusa 6c, *every 2–3 hours*.
- Convulsions during teething, with drawing backward of the head.
  Cicuta 6c, *every 2–3 hours*.
- As a general treatment, in children prone to convulsions.
  Mag phos 6x and **Calc phos 6x**, *two tissue salts, twice a day for 1 month*.

Cradle Cap

Cradle cap is more properly known as seborrheic eczema. It is a scurfy accumulation of skin, most commonly on the scalp, but can also affect the face, neck, armpit or loins. The skin can become yellow and soggy looking, although it can often be lifted by applying olive oil. The affected area should be kept clean, with regular washing after olive oil applications. After washing, apply **Calendula** tincture, diluted 1 in 10, and allow to dry.

TREATMENT

- Cradle cap, with white chalk-like crust.
  Calc carb 6c, every 2–3 hours.
- Crusting lesions through the hair.
  Calc carb 6c, every 2–3 hours.
- For crusty lesions around the hair line.
  Nat mur 6x, a tissue salt, every 2–3 hours.
- Skin dry and scaly, but not infected.
  Lycopodium 6c, every 3–4 hours.

- Skin crusty, can weep or ooze straw-colored fluid. Can crack and bleed.
  Graphites 6c, every 3–4 hours.
- Affecting mainly the face and scalp, lesions thickly encrusted, with swollen glands.
  Viola 6c, every 3–4 hours.
- Scabby patches on the scalp, which ooze and mat the hair together.
  Vinca 6c, every 3–4 hours.

Crying and Irritability

A baby's way of communicating a variety of complaints—hunger, thirst, discomfort, pain, boredom, loneliness, or anxiety—shows this common pattern. Irritability and crying is probably never without a cause, but the cause can be quite difficult to find. It may be something as minor as clothing that is uncomfortable, or being hungry; it may be an episode of teething or colic coming on.

If the baby has a fever, looks ill, or is continually distressed, then remedies can be used while the condition is watched closely. Failure to improve warrants professional attention. A unusually high-pitched cry, coupled with vomiting and intolerance of light, may indicate meningitis, a serious condition requiring immediate allopathic treatment.

TREATMENT

- Irritable, restless and demanding. Wants to be held, hard to please.
  Chamomilla 6c, every 1–2 hours.
- Irritable and changeable, always better from being carried or held.
  Pulsatilla 6c, every 1–2 hours.
- Irritability with anger. Spiteful, does not invite comfort. Particularly during teething, or if there are boils or styes.
  Staphysagria 6c, every 1–2 hours.

- Irritability with anger, better from warmth. May have constipation or diarrhea.
  Nux vomica 6c, every 1–2 hours.
- Complaining child, worse from comfort, often with white tongue.
  Ant crud 6c, every 1–2 hours.
- Child is anxious in sleep, restless dreams with half-opened eyes.
  Chamomilla 6c, every 2–3 hours.

$\mathcal{D}$*elivery*

Being a natural process, birth is usually problem-free. However after a difficult birth, a long or very rapid labor, or when forceps have been used, a number of remedies are useful to comfort the baby, although in serious cases allopathic advice should be sought.

TREATMENT

- Baby shocked, frightened and anxious.
  Aconite 6c, every 30–60 minutes.
- Baby is pale, breathless, gasping, suffocated.
  Ant tart 6c, every 30–60 minutes.

- Baby pale, collapsed and cold.
  Carbo veg 6c, every 30–60 minutes.
- Bruised head or purple marks after birth.
  Arnica 6c, 1 dose per day.

Diaper Rash

Diaper rash is usually seen as sore, red, scalded skin around the genitals and buttocks, often from leaving diapers on overly long, or from chemical residues left in the diaper after washing. It can be improved by allowing the skin to dry as much as possible, preferably in the open air. **Chickweed** ointment, or Penaten cream from a pharmacy, can then be applied to soothe the skin. Diapers should be rinsed one extra time. Avoid the use of plastic coverings as they do not allow the skin to breathe.

TREATMENT

- Diaper rash, with red skin worse from heat and bathing, better in warm air.
  Sulphur 6c, every 2–3 hours.
- Diaper rash in chubby babies, sweaty around the head.
  Calc carb 6c, every 2–3 hours.

- Diaper rash from scalding urine, irritating the skin.
  Medorrhinum 30c, 1 dose a day for 3 days.

Diarrhea

Diarrhea in infants is potentially dangerous, as it can lead to dehydration quite quickly. The symptoms of dehydration are dry mouth, sunken eyes and depressed fontanels. To keep the infant's fluid intake up give water with a mixture of special salts (Gastrolyte) added, as well as the usual feeds. If diarrhea persists for longer than 12 hours in infants, or the stools are bloody, allopathic advice should be sought.

TREATMENT

- Diarrhea after exposure to cold winds, with restlessness and anxiety.
  Aconite 6c, every 2–3 hours.

- Greenish stools, especially with vomiting of milk.
  Aethusa 6c, every 2–3 hours.

- Watery, green stool, in crying, fretful baby, wanting to be held.
  Chamomilla 6c, every 2–3 hours.
- Diarrhea in babies who do not tolerate milk well. Stool is watery, green and frothy, and the child has an acid odor.
  Mag carb 6c, every 3–4 hours.
- Sour-smelling or offensive stool, with salivation and great straining.
  Mercurius 6c, every 2–3 hours.
- Offensive, fermented, painful stool, with vomiting, and pale face.
  Ipecac 6c, every 2–3 hours.
- Stools fermented, foamy, like yeast; grass-green, mucous or watery.
  Ipecac 6c, every 2–3 hours.
- Diarrhea in children while feeding or teething: profuse and offensive, green, watery and gushing.
  Podophyllum 6c, every 2–3 hours.
- Watery, painless diarrhea, with wind and undigested milk in the stools.
  China 6c, every 2–3 hours.
- Diarrhea with abdominal distension, rumbling and wind. Hungry but no appetite.
  China 6c, every 2–3 hours.
- Diarrhea caused by overfeeding.
  Nux vomica 6c, every 2–3 hours.
- Slightest movement brings on diarrhea.
  Bryonia 6c, every 2–3 hours.

Hiccup

Hiccup is a spasmodic contraction of the diaphragm that closes the throat, resulting in a sudden shutting off of breath. It usually passes quite quickly, although persistent hiccups can be distressing and exhausting.

TREATMENT

- Spasmodic attacks, better by pressure and warmth. Mag phos is the principal remedy.
  Mag phos 6x, a tissue salt, every 1–2 hours.
- With irritability and restlessness.
  Chamomilla 6c, every 2–3 hours.
- Hiccups that bring up sour, bitter wind.
  Dioscorea 6c, every 2–3 hours.

Jaundice

Jaundice is the appearance of a yellowish pigment in the skin. It appears in mild form on the second or third day after birth due to immaturity of the liver, and fades a few days later. It is improved by exposing the child to fluorescent light or sunlight, although you should be careful of glare and sunburn. The child should be given plenty to drink to flush out excess pigment. If jaundice persists or deepens after the appropriate remedies are used, allopathic advice should be sought.

TREATMENT

- In the usual case, to hasten disappearance.
  China 6c, twice daily for a few days.
- Baby is irritable, thirsty and hot.
  Chamomilla 6c, twice daily for a few days.
- Baby is irritable, with constipation.
  Nux vomica 6c, twice daily for a few days.

- If Chamomilla is not effective and symptoms persist.
  Mercurius 6c, twice daily for a few days.
- If jaundice is due to Rhesus incompatibility.
  Crotalus 6c, twice daily.

Milk Crust

This skin disorder shows as clusters of small white pustules on a red surface, appearing first on the face and spreading from there over the whole body. In a short time they can burst and form thin yellow crusts. The lesions can itch considerably, and the baby can be restless and fretful. Applying **Calendula** ointment or **Chickweed** ointment will assist healing and keep the skin soft. **Solanum nigrum** ointment should be used in resistant cases.

TREATMENT

- In the early stages, where the eruption is red and inflamed, and the baby is restless and anxious.
  Aconite 6c, every 2–3 hours.
- When pustules form and the rash spreads.
  Rhus tox 6c, every 2–3 hours.
- In entrenched cases, with cracking.
  Viola 6c, every 2–3 hours.

- Lesions of the scalp producing a white deposit looking like chalk.
  Calc carb 6c, every 3–4 hours.
- Lesions particularly affecting the fingers and palms of the hands.
  Anagallis 6c, every 3–4 hours.
- Small vesicles, like blisters, around the hair line.
  Nat mur 6x, a tissue salt, every 2–3 hours.

Prickly Heat

Prickly heat shows as itchy red pimples during hot periods. The skin should be kept as dry as possible; in irritated conditions **Chickweed** ointment, or Penaten cream from a pharmacy, can be applied.

TREATMENT

- Prickly heat, with irritability and restlessness.
  Chamomilla 6c, every 2–3 hours.
- Prickly heat, worse from bathing, particularly in hot water.
  Sulphur 6c, every 2–3 hours.

- Prickly heat, with restlessness and small blisters like pinheads.
  Rhus tox 6c, every 2–3 hours.
- Itching violently at night.
  Juglans regia 6c, every 2–3 hours.

Snuffles

Snuffles are due to a thickening of the mucous membrane lining the nose, making breathing through the nose difficult. It would not be particularly noticeable in older children, but it prevents babies feeding.

TREATMENT

- Complete blockage of the nose, but little or no discharge.
  Sambucus 6c, *every 2–3 hours*.
- Nose runs during the day but is dry and obstructed at night.
  Nux vomica 6c, *every 2–3 hours*.

- With irritability and running of watery mucus from the nose.
  Chamomilla 6c, *every 2–3 hours*.
- Discharge green–yellow, comes and goes.
  Pulsatilla 6c, *every 2–3 hours*.

Teething

The first teeth appear at about 6–10 months, and the last at about 20 months. During this period most babies will suffer discomfort, and often find relief by chewing on teething rings or zweiback. Allowing the baby to chew on a piece of ice is often beneficial. There is usually salivation, often diarrhea, and frequently irritability. Catnip or chamomile tea is a useful drink for babies at this time: it soothes and slightly sedates. Clove oil may also be rubbed on the gums.

TREATMENT

- Swollen tender gums, with salivation, restlessness and irritability. Child wants to be held; may have one cheek red, the other pale. Particularly if there is green diarrhea.
  Chamomilla 6c, *every 1–2 hours*.
- As a general remedy in chubby, sweaty babies, smelling sour.
  Calc carb 6c, *every 2–3 hours*.
- Irresistible desire to bite the teeth together. Teeth clenched, or biting on everything.
  Phytolacca 6c, *every 2–3 hours*.

- Great desire to press the gums together, with hot glowing cheeks and often a gushing diarrhea.
  Podophyllum 6c, *every 2–3 hours*.
- Teething trouble in chilly, dark and wiry babies.
  Calc phos 6x, *a tissue salt, every 2–3 hours*.
- Head flushed and hot, rolling from side to side. Restless; may be delirious or have convulsions.
  Belladonna 6c, *every 1–2 hours*.

- Convulsions during teething, arching backwards.
  Cicuta 6c, every 2–3 hours.
- Vomiting during teething, bringing up food with great force.
  Aethusa 6c, every 2–3 hours.

- Teething with mouth ulcers.
  Borax 6c, every 3–4 hours.
- Teeth decay almost as soon as they are through.
  Staphysagria 6c, morning and evening for a few weeks.

Thrush

Thrush is due to the overgrowth of the fungus *Candida albicans*. It commonly appears as white patches on the tongues of nursing infants, and looks like milk curds, although it will not brush off. Usually it runs a course of about two weeks, but is dangerous if it spreads to other areas. It often follows treatment by antibiotics.

TREATMENT

- Whitish or yellowish patches, joining together.
  Sulphuric acid 6c, every 2–3 hours.
- Thick tongue, with yellow–white deposit.
  Mercurius 6c, every 2–3 hours.

- In resistant cases, especially with ulceration.
  Borax 6c, every 2–3 hours.

Vomiting

Bringing up small amounts of food is common in infants, but if nearly all the food is vomited for more than 24 hours, allopathic advice should be sought. Repeated vomiting is very dehydrating for a young baby: symptoms of dehydration are dry mouth, sunken eyes and depressed areas of the skull. Replace fluids if necessary with water to which salts (Gastrolyte) have been added. There may be obstruction of the intestine if the vomiting is accompanied by bouts of screaming, or if the vomit is greenish–yellow, and allopathic advice should then be sought immediately.

- Milk is vomited with great force as soon as swallowed, followed by distress and exhaustion.
  Aethusa 6c, every 2–3 hours.
- Milk stays down for a time, but reappears as sour green or yellow curds, large and profuse.
  Aethusa 6c, every 2–3 hours.
- Sudden vomiting of milk, with oily sweat and irritability.
  Mercurius 6c, every 3–4 hours.
- Feverish and irritable, with one cheek red, one pale, wants to be carried.
  Chamomilla 6c, every 1–2 hours.
- Restless and changeable, wanting to be picked up.
  Pulsatilla 6c, every 2–3 hours.
- Vomiting of milk followed by retching.
  Ipecac 6c, every 2–3 hours.

- Vomiting with constipation, stools dry and crumbly.
  Mag carb 6c, every 2–3 hours.
- Vomiting with stomach full of wind and rumbling, obviously painful.
  Nat carb 6c, every 2–3 hours.
- Vomiting without crying. Waxy pallor and bluish rings around eyes.
  Phos ac 6c, every 2–3 hours.
- Vomiting in a baby with sour head, sweats during sleep.
  Calc carb 6c, every 2–3 hours.
- Vomiting with marked distension of the abdomen.
  Lac caninum 6c, every 2–3 hours.
- Vomiting in a tense baby, especially troubled by hiccups.
  Mag phos 6x, a tissue salt, every 2–3 hours.

6

The Treatment
of Children

Adenoids

The adenoids are lymphatic glands behind the nose, which can enlarge and cause obstruction of the nose, throat and eustachian tubes in the ear. This often shows as mouth breathing, because of the partially blocked nose, and nasal-sounding speech. Food allergies are commonly a primary cause, and should be investigated to resolve the problem.

TREATMENT

- Enlarged adenoids after vaccination, especially in children with profuse foot sweats.
  Silicea 6x, a tissue salt, every 3–4 hours.
- Enlarged adenoids in slow-growing children, with easy fatigue.
  Calc phos 6x, a tissue salt, every 3–4 hours.

- Enlarged adenoids in pale, overweight children, prone to head sweats at night.
  Calc carb 6c, every 3–4 hours.
- Enlarged adenoids in children with yellow nasal discharge, thick and bland, worse in a warm room and flowing freely outdoors.
  Pulsatilla 6c, every 3–4 hours.

Bed Wetting

Bed wetting in the normal case occurs less and less after the age of two. However about 10 per cent of four- and five-year-olds regularly bed wet, and a further 10 per cent do so on occasion. Causes include anxiety, problems in the family and at school, food allergies, acidic urine, urinary infections and worms.

TREATMENT

The following remedies have a good history of success.

- Large quantities of urine, soaking the bed.
  Plantago 6c, morning and evening.
- Wetting during dreams, soaking the bed.
  Equisetum 6c, morning and evening.
- Soaks the bed later in sleep, anxious and irritable.
  Lycopodium 6c, morning and evening.
- Bed wetting during the first sleep, especially if there are frequent nightmares.
  Belladonna 6c, morning and evening.
- Bed wetting in young children and old people.
  Calc phos 6x, a tissue salt, morning and evening.
- Child sleeps deeply, cannot wake fast enough to get to toilet.
  Kreosotum 6c, morning and evening.
- Wets both day and night, leaks when coughing, sneezing, or laughing. Wets early in the night, unaware of passing urine.
  Causticum 6c, morning and evening.
- Bed wetting in older children, from nervousness or lack of nerve power.
  Kali phos 6x, a tissue salt, morning and evening.
- Bed wetting in children, with excessive flow of watery urine.
  Nat mur 6x, a tissue salt, morning and evening.

Chickenpox

Chickenpox is otherwise known as varicella, a viral disease, and is characterised by fever followed by a rash. It has an incubation period of about 14 days and is contagious until the scabs form. The disorder starts as a chill, followed by fever, aching of the back and legs, and loss of appetite. Vomiting may occur. On the second day the rash shows as more or less transparent vesicles, which begin as a pink dot then blister to the size of a pea. The spots first appear on the trunk, then spread to the face and limbs; within 24 hours after appearance they become pustular, and after a few days dry up to form scabs which scale off within a week. At this stage the disease is no longer infectious. Serious complications are rare; the most usual is secondary infection of the lesions. More serious complications are encephalomyelitis, pneumonia and myocarditis.

TREATMENT

- For general protection of family and friends.
  Varicella 30c, once daily for 7 days.
- For the fever, in the initial stages, and to abort the illness.
  Ferrum phos 6x, a tissue salt, every 2–3 hours.

When the rash appears
- Clear vesicles with a dry and itchy base, aggravated by scratching.
  Rhus tox 6c, every 3–4 hours, is often the only remedy needed.
- Scaly, pustular burning and itching eruption, worse at night.
  Ant crud 6c, every 3–4 hours.
- Vesicles with white pus.
  Kali mur 6x, a tissue salt, every 3–4 hours.

- If the fever is accompanied by anxiety and restlessness.
  Aconite 6c, every 1–2 hours.
- Fever with flushed face, enlarged pupils, glassy eyes and restless delirium.
  Belladonna 6c, every 2–3 hours.

- For lesions that are very large, with drowsiness and sweat.
  Ant tart 6c, every 3–4 hours.
- Vesicles with yellow pus and dry, scaly skin.
  Kali sulph 6x, a tissue salt, every 3–4 hours.
- During convalescence, to assist recovery.
  Calc phos 6x, a tissue salt, every 3–4 hours.

Croup

Croup usually starts as a mild respiratory disorder, with some hoarseness. It develops quickly, typically at night, with a sensation of suffocation, a husky voice, and the characteristic crowing, barking cough. It is often difficult to breathe in, resulting in substantial anxiety and fear. The attack can last from a few minutes to a few hours, and may recur for a few nights.

TREATMENT

Treatment should begin with using a steadily steaming kettle to humidify the room (you can use an electric frypan, or even turn on all the hot faucets in the bathroom to fill the room with steam), and the concurrent use of homeopathic remedies usually affords a rapid resolution.

- Anxious suffocative attacks, with dry cough and restlessness. Head is hot, body is cold.
  Aconite 6c, every 3–4 hours.
- Deep, dull and whistling cough, or loose, thick, wheezing and rattling, with feeling of needles in the throat, better from humid air.
  Hepar sulph 6c, every 3–4 hours.

- Deep, dry, hollow barking, with construction and painful soreness and burning of the chest.
  Spongia 6c, every 3–4 hours.
- In desperate cases.
  Lachesis 30c, one dose.

Earache

Ears should always be treated with care, and should not be poked. Any wax in the ear can be cleared by running warmed olive oil gently into the canal, until it is full. The oil should be kept in the ear for about ten minutes, then allowed to run out. Insects and other objects may also be cleared using this method. Do not attempt to clear wax during an infection.

Home homeopathic treatment of earache should be approached with caution, as infection can cause scarring and serious damage to the hearing if left untreated. As a general rule, homeopathic treatment should only be used in uncomplicated earache, when there is inflammation but no evidence of discharge. In these cases, or when the earache is recurrent, these remedies can be used while professional advice is being sought. About one-third of earaches in children are due to teething.

TREATMENT

- The child is irritable, anxious and restless, with burning pain.
  Aconite 6c, every 30–60 minutes.
- Earache with fever, red ear, heat and throbbing. Child is restless, flushed, and sensitive to noise, movement and touch.
  Belladonna 6c, every 30–60 minutes.
- Child is restless, irritable and thirsty, wanting to be held constantly. Pain is worse between 9 p.m. and midnight.
  Chamomilla 6c, every 30–60 minutes.
- Fever, pain and congested face, or flushing, with alternate pallor and redness, occasionally with nosebleed.
  Ferrum phos 6x, a tissue salt, every 30–60 minutes.
- Earache with sharp neuralgic pains in or around the ear.
  Mag phos 6x, a tissue salt, every 3–4 hours.
- Child is irritable, changeable and restless, demands company and prefers open air.
  Pulsatilla 6c, every 30–60 minutes.

- Earache with swelling of the glands and tongue coated white.
  Kali mur 6x, a tissue salt, every 3–4 hours.
- Earache with yellow catarrh of the ear and yellow tongue.
  Kali sulph 6x, a tissue salt, every 3–4 hours.
- Child is tearful and seeks comfort, but not irritable. Pain centers behind the ear, is sensitive to touch, shooting and burning, and is made better by hot applications.
  Capsicum 6c, every 30–60 minutes.
- Pains are burning and worse between midnight and 3 a.m., better by hot applications.
  Arsenicum 6c, every 3–4 hours.
- Shooting pains in the ears.
  Hypericum 6c, every 30–60 minutes.
- Pain is stinging and burning, better by cold applications.
  Apis 6c, every 30–60 minutes.
- Deafness, with noises in the ear, from nervous weakness or exhaustion.
  Kali phos 6x, a tissue salt, every 3–4 hours.

Glue Ear

Glue ear is the name given to an accumulation of thick waxy exudate in the middle ear, common in children. It reduces hearing ability, and may often make the voice reverberate. There is usually no pain and no infection. While the wax may be cleared using warm olive oil, it is important that the cause is treated, as it can make ear infections more likely. Food allergies are often the primary cause, and should be investigated to resolve the problem. Surgery to insert grommets can usually be avoided.

TREATMENT

- Intermittent deafness, mouth breathing, yellow–green mucus from the nose. Child complains, wants comfort and consolation, is very changeable.
  Pulsatilla 6c, every 3–4 hours.
- Enlarged glands with catarrhal discharges in sweaty children, with cracking noises.
  Calc carb 6c, every 3–4 hours.

- Deafness, caused by swelling of the eustachian tubes or catarrhal accumulation.
  Kali mur 6x, a tissue salt, every 3–4 hours.
- Thick, smelly, discharge from outer ear, with copious production of saliva during sleep.
  Mercurius 6c, every 3–4 hours.

Fever

Fever is not an enemy to be suppressed, but a signal that the body is working properly in an attempt to ward off an invader. Fevers are generally preceded by chilliness, and there may be headache and a feeling of weakness in the limbs. There is usually a hot stage, where the skin feels dry; there is an increase in pulse rate, excessive thirst and no appetite.

Mild fevers are generally regarded as above the normal body temperature of 98.6°F (36–37°C) but below 100°F (38°C), moderate fevers as 100°–103°F (38–39.5°C) and high fevers as over 104°F (40°C). Dosing with paracetamol or aspirin may bring the temperature down for a while, but will not assist the germ-fighting process, and may even lead to complications. If treated early using homeopathic medicines, fevers usually improve and rarely worsen. However any fever over 104°F (40°C), or showing symptoms of breathing difficulties, convulsions, turning blue around the lips or vomiting, is to be regarded seriously and allopathic advice should be sought.

Fever can take one of two forms homeopathically, depending on the speed of onset, gradual or sudden.

TREATMENT

A fever of sudden onset

- Early stages of any fever, with excessive thirst not relieved by drinking, and dry skin.
  Nat mur 6x, a tissue salt, every 1–2 hours.

- Sudden fever, often around midnight or after cold, dry weather, with pale face, anxiety and thirst.
  Aconite 6c, every 1–2 hours.

- Sudden rise in temperature with red, congested face, pounding pulse, staring eyes, restlessness and delirium.
  Belladonna 6c, every 1–2 hours.

- Fever with swelling of the throat. Sharp, stinging pains. Feels chilly despite fever, has no thirst, feels worse in hot rooms.
  Apis 6c, every 1–2 hours.

A fever of gradual onset

- Face alternately red and pale, feels shivery in spite of frequent sweats, throbbing headache improved by cool applications. Skin is moist, tongue red and shiny.
  Ferrum phos 6x, a tissue salt, every 1–2 hours.

- Second stage of any fever, with gray–white coating on the tongue.
  Kali mur 6x, a tissue salt, every 1–2 hours.

- Feverish, irritable and restless, craves heat. Thirsty, but drinking cold water brings on chills.
  Nux vomica 6c, every 3–4 hours.

- High fever with aching muscles, weakness, heaviness and trembling of the limbs. Looks sleepy, has no thirst.
  Gelsemium 6c, every 2–3 hours.

- Feverish, irritable and sweating, dry mouth, with great thirst at long intervals, wants to lie still and be left alone.
  Bryonia 6c, every 2–3 hours.

- Fever worse between midnight and 3 a.m., child restless, anxious and exhausted, chilly, thirsty for small sips of water, with burning pains better by heat.
  Arsenicum alb 6c, every 2–3 hours.
- Feels worse for changes in temperature; breath is offensive, body has fetid odor and greasy sweat. Moist mouth yet intense thirst.
  Mercurius 6c, every 2–3 hours.

- Exhausted and restless, shivers and sweats profusely.
  Rhus tox 6c, every 2–3 hours.
- Child craves cold drinks, which are vomited as soon as taken.
  Phosphorus 6c, every 2–3 hours.
- Fever that comes on in the evening, with hot, dry skin.
  Kali sulph 6c, a tissue salt, every 1–2 hours.

German Measles

German measles, otherwise known as rubella, is a mild but very infectious viral disease, with an incubation period of about 18 days. It is contagious from the first appearance of symptoms until the rash disappears, usually three or four days. It is similar to measles but is more trivial. One attack usually confers immunity for life. The lesions are paler, completely flat, and do not usually run together. The first symptoms are a slight cold, some fever and a sore throat. The lymph nodes behind the ears and at the back of the neck may swell. The rash is orange–red, appears first on the face and scalp, and spreads to the body and arms the same day. The rash fades after two or three days. Complications are rare in children, but dangerous in pregnant women, as they can cause heart defect, cataract, mental retardation and deafness in the fetus.

TREATMENT

To treat the illness in the fever stage, to limit the course of the disease, see Fever. Here are some common remedies for fever.

- As a prophylactic to reduce duration and severity, for family and friends.
  Rubella 30c, once daily for 7 days.

- Sudden fever often around midnight or after cold, dry weather, with pale face, anxiety and thirst.
  Aconite 6c, every 1–2 hours.

- Face alternately red and pale, feels shivery in spite of frequent sweats, throbbing headache improved by cool applications. Skin is moist, tongue red and shiny.
  Ferrum phos 6x, *a tissue salt, every 1–2 hours.*

- Sudden rise in temperature with red, congested face, pounding pulse, staring eyes, restlessness and delirium.
  Belladonna 6c, *every 1–2 hours.*

When the rash appears

- Measles-like eruptions, changeable, tearful, restless and irritable, wanting to be held.
  Pulsatilla 6c, *every 3–4 hours.*
- If the spots coalesce, producing a scarlatina-type appearance.
  Belladonna 6c, *every 3–4 hours.*

- Swollen glands, ear pains on swallowing, symptoms alleviated by cold drinks.
  Phytolacca 6c, *every 3–4 hours.*

Impetigo

Impetigo is otherwise known as school sores, and is an infectious skin eruption with pustules and crusts, usually around the mouth and the lower half of the face. It is most common in children, although adults can contract it also. It begins as clear vesicles, which soon become cloudy, rupture and spread, and begin to crust over. Bacteria are spread by touching the blisters, then touching another part of the body, or by using contaminated towels or linen. It is most serious in newborn babies, where the bacteria may spread to the kidneys: failure to resolve in the newborn warrants immediate allopathic treatment.

TREATMENT

Bathe the affected areas morning and evening with **Hypercal** (equal parts of Calendula tincture and Hypericum tincture), diluted 1 in 10. When dry apply **Solanum nigrum** ointment to the lesions.

- As a prophylactic to reduce duration and severity, for family and friends.
  Strep/Staph 30c, once daily for 7 days
- Lesions with splinter-like pains, very sensitive to draughts and even the slightest touch.
  Hepar sulph 6c, every 3–4 hours.
- Thick, yellow, spreading crusts, with white-coated tongue and blisters around the nostrils and mouth.
  Ant crud 6c, every 3–4 hours.
- Pustules on an inflamed base, itching, stinging and oozing pus. Scrotum most affected.
  Croton tig 6c, every 3–4 hours.
- Eruptions in clusters, with violent burning and itching, stinging and tingling.
  Rhus tox 6c, every 3–4 hours.
- Eruptions ulcerate and form thick suppurating crusts, especially on the scalp, oozing pus that irritates surrounding skin.
  Mezereum 6c, every 3–4 hours.
- Humid eruptions turning into thick, yellow–brown crusts, itching and bleeding when scratched.
  Dulcamara 6c, every 3–4 hours.
- Yellowish-brown crusts, itching from the warmth of the bed, with offensive breath, oily sweat.
  Mercurius 6c, every 3–4 hours.
- Entrenched cases, with much pus and failure to heal.
  Calc sulph 6x, a tissue salt, every 3–4 hours.

Irritability

Like crying in babies, it is unlikely that irritability in small children occurs without a reason, but its cause may be obscure. A few minutes of close attention and communication may do more than any remedy, but a number have had good results.

TREATMENT

- Irritable and changeable, always better from being carried or held.
  Pulsatilla 6c, every 3–4 hours.
- Complaining child, worse from comfort, often with white tongue.
  Ant crud 6c, every 3–4 hours.

- Crying or whining without apparent cause. Hard to please: wants this and that, which is then refused. Restless, thirsty, wants to be carried out, but no better from it.
  Chamomilla 6c, every 1–2 hours.
- Irritability with anger, worse in mornings, better from warmth. May have constipation or diarrhea.
  Nux vomica 6c, every 3–4 hours.
- Child is anxious in sleep, restless dreams with half-opened eyes, irritable on waking.
  Chamomilla 6c, every 1–2 hours.
- Irritability with anger. Spiteful, does not invite comfort. Particularly during teething, or if there is a history of boils or styes.
  Staphysagria 6c, every 3–4 hours.
- Wants things, but rejects when offered, with irritability. Appetite can be variable, or always hungry.
  Cina 6c, every 3–4 hours.
- As a result of fussing.
  Hepar sulph 6c, every 3–4 hours.
- After rich food.
  Nux vomica 6c, every 3–4 hours.

Measles

Measles, otherwise known as morbillis, is a highly infectious viral disease. It has an incubation period of 7–14 days, average about 11. It is contagious for four days before the appearance of the rash, and until it fades. In the early stages it has the symptoms of influenza: there is inflammation and fever accompanied by sneezing, drowsiness, lassitude, irritability, aching in the back and limbs, shivering and thirst. There is a peculiar, hoarse, dry cough.

The measles eruption appears generally on the fourth day, with small red spots like fleabites joining together into irregular circles as horseshoes. The spots are elevated, and may take 1–2 days to mature; they are usually first seen at the back of the ears and frontal hairline. At this stage the fever and respiratory symptoms will be at their height.

At 7–8 days from the onset, the illness subsides and the eruption fades, replaced by small bran-like scales, lasting about a further week. During this period, it is important that there is no exposure to chill or cold, and that exposure to bright light is minimised.

Most cases are uncomplicated, the most common complication being convulsion in young children when the rash is appearing. Conjunctivitis, ear inflammation, bronchitis, pneumonia, gastroenteritis, appendicitis and encephalomyelitis may also occur. Measles is more serious in adults than in children, although one infection usually confers life immunity.

Treatment in the early stages is the same as for fever and influenza, and well-chosen remedies can abort the progress of the illness at this early stage. In the later stages the following remedies are valuable. If complications develop in spite of the use of well-chosen remedies, particularly earache, or if fever persists after the rash begins to fade, allopathic advice should be sought.

TREATMENT

■ As general protection for family and friends.

Morbillinum 30c, once daily for 7 days.

To treat the illness in the fever stage and to limit the course of the disease, see Fever. Here are some common remedies for fever.

■ Sudden fever, often around midnight or after cold dry weather, with pale face, anxiety and thirst.
Aconite 6c, every 1–2 hours.

■ Sudden rise in temperature with red, congested face, pounding pulse, staring eyes, restlessness and delirium.
Belladonna 6c, every 1–2 hours.

■ Face alternately red and pale, feels shivery in spite of frequent sweats, throbbing headache improved by cool applications. Skin is moist, tongue red and shiny.
Ferrum phos 6x, a tissue salt, every 1–2 hours.

When the rash has appeared

■ Child restless, peevish and seeking comfort, with large pustules.
Pulsatilla 6c, every 3–4 hours.

■ Rash with hard, dry and painful cough, always worse from movement.
Bryonia 6c, every 3–4 hours.

■ Itchy rash and peeling of the skin in fine, dry scales.
Kali sulph 6x, a tissue salt, every 3–4 hours.

■ Tight, dry cough, with thirst for cold drinks and perhaps vomiting.
Phosphorus 6c, every 3–4 hours.

- In the later stages, with headache, eyes red and streaming, nose watering.
  Euphrasia 6c, every 3–4 hours.
- Measles with purplish appearance. Convalescence slow, and patient weak and prostrate.
  Sulphur 6c, every 3–4 hours.

- To strengthen the constitution during convalescence.
  Calc phos 6x, a tissue salt, every 3–4 hours.

Mumps

Mumps is otherwise known as parotiditis. This common childhood viral disease has swelling of the glands instead of a rash. The incubation period is usually 18 days, although it may vary from 12 to 26. The disease is contagious in the infected person from 1–2 days before symptoms appear until 1–2 days after they disappear.

Often the first noticeable symptom is a painful swelling of the parotid glands on the side of the neck. Either or both sides can be affected. The swelling increases for 2–3 days, accompanied by fever, loss of appetite, headache and back pain, and subsides within 10 days.

Complications are rare, and include inflammation of the testicle in the male, and ovarian and breast involvement in the female. Inflammation of the brain is an occasional complication, with dizziness, vomiting and headache. Pancreas inflammation may also occur. If the child develops severe headache, shrinks away from bright light, or is stupid or drowsy, allopathic advice should be sought.

TREATMENT

- As general protection for family and friends.
  Parotidinum 30c, once daily for 7 days.

- Child flushed, eyes staring and glassy. The glands are swollen, hot, red and sensitive to pressure. The pains are shooting, extending to the ear.
  Belladonna 6c, every 3–4 hours.

- Swollen glands, offensive salivation, foul tongue and offensive sweat.
  Mercurius 6c, *every 3–4 hours.*
- Glands highly inflamed and enlarged, with restlessness.
  Rhus tox 6c, *every 3–4 hours.*
- Glands swollen and stony hard, with ear pains on swallowing.
  Phytolacca 6c, *every 3–4 hours.*
- For glandular swelling, pain on swallowing and a white-coated tongue.
  Kali mur 6c, *a tissue salt, every 3–4 hours.*
- Face is pale and cold, but the patient craves fresh air.
  Carbo veg 6c, *every 3–4 hours.*
- If the swelling subsides, to be followed by throbbing headache.
  Belladonna 6c, *every 3–4 hours.*

- Severe headache, in the established stage. Saliva thick and sticky.
  Pilocarpine mur 6c, *every 3–4 hours.*
- If the breasts or testicles become involved.
  Pulsatilla 6c, *every 3–4 hours.*
- Pale, cold face, and involvement of breasts or testes.
  Carbo veg 6c, *every 3–4 hours.*
- If the patient gets a cold, with yellow discharge.
  Pulsatilla 6c, *every 3–4 hours.*
- In cases of complication, with pancreas inflammation.
  Phosphorus 6c, *every 3–4 hours.*
- During convalescence, to restore strength and vitality.
  Calc phos 6x, *a tissue salt, every 3–4 hours.*

Nosebleeds

The immediate treatment for a nosebleed is to sit the patient upright, and apply cold water or ice to the root of the nose to stop bleeding. The nose should not be blown, and can be pinched at the soft part near the root to constrict the blood vessels. Excessive bleeding after a blow, or bleeding that does not cease, should receive allopathic examination.

TREATMENT

- As a local application, on small plugs of cotton wool inserted into the nostrils to arrest bleeding.
  Hamamelis tincture.

- Red face, nose red and swollen, with throbbing.
  Belladonna 6c, *every 1–2 hours.*

- Small amounts of bright blood whenever nose is blown.
  Phosphorus 6c, *every 1–2 hours.*
- Simple nosebleeds, with profuse red blood, with pain from eyes to root of the nose.
  Millefolium 6c, *every 3–4 hours.*

- Recurrent bleeding without obvious cause, especially in pale, sensitive children.
  Ferrum phos 6x, *a tissue salt, every 1–2 hours.*

Scarlet Fever

Scarlet fever is otherwise known as scarlatina. It is a bacterial (streptococcal) disease and it has an incubation period of 1–7 days, average 2–5. The active stage is over as soon as the fever is gone—usually about seven days. The disease is most common in late winter and early spring.

Symptoms vary a great deal, from nothing but a sore throat and swelling of the lymph nodes of the neck, to fever with purulent exudation from the tonsils, nausea, vomiting and headache. The bright red rash usually appears on the second day, first behind the ears, and rapidly spreads, being most intense in the folds of the arms and legs. The face is not affected by the rash, although it is usually flushed, and the region around the mouth is pale. The tongue shows a characteristic strawberry appearance, usually furred. The rash usually fades after 7 days, and the skin peels, especially on the palms and soles. Complications are rare, but include suppurative earache, sinusitis and suppuration of the lymph glands of the neck.

TREATMENT

- As a prophylactic to reduce duration and severity, for family and friends.
  Scarlatinum 30c, *one dose per day for 7 days*, or *Streptococcin 30c*, *one dose per day during the outbreak.*

- Face is flushed and feverish, with pallor around the mouth. Belladonna is often the only remedy needed.
  Belladonna 6c, *every 3–4 hours.*

- Profuse salivation, with offensive mouth and sore throat. Chills alternate with fever.
  Mercurius 6c, every 3–4 hours.

- For suppuration afterwards.
  Mercurius 6c, every 3–4 hours.
- Skin comes off in fine powdery scales.
  Arsenicum 6c, every 3–4 hours.

Sleep Problems

Disturbed sleep in small children is often the result of another ailment—teething or a cold virus, for instance. Some children, however, seem to have permanently poor sleeping habits, and the following remedies may be of use in such cases.

TREATMENT

- Sleepy but cannot get to sleep.
  Chamomilla 6c, every 2–3 hours.
- Child sleeps on stomach, grinds teeth and jerks violently during sleep, wakes in a fright, may suffer from worms.
  Cina 6c, every 3–4 hours.
- Child sleeps with eyes open, moans during sleep, irritable and impossible to please when awake.
  Chamomilla 6c, every 2–3 hours.
- Child sleeps lightly, jerks in sleep. Disturbed sleep after emotional upsets.
  Ignatia 6c, every 3–4 hours.

- Child starts and cries out in anxiety during sleep, has head sweats.
  Calc carb 6c, every 3–4 hours.
- Child sleeps for short periods only, moans during sleep.
  Ant tart 6c, every 3–4 hours.
- Sleepwalking, in thin children with large heads.
  Silicea 6x, a tissue salt, every 3–4 hours.
- Nightmares in sensitive child, weeps and screams, or fear of dark.
  Phosphorus 6c, every 3–4 hours.
- Night terrors in children, sleepwalking, fidgety hands.
  Kali brom 6c, every 3–4 hours.

Whooping Cough

Whooping cough is a highly infectious disease, serious in very young children, and occasionally fatal in babies. The incubation period for whooping cough is 1–2 weeks, and the disorder is infectious for up to three weeks after the onset. It can last for anything from 2–10 weeks. It starts like a cold, with a mild fever and runny nose, but the harsh, dry coughs become grouped together progressively into spasms of coughing. A whoop develops at the end of a coughing spasm, as the child fights to regain breath. Coughing may be violent enough to cause blue face, nosebleeds and vomiting. Complications include pneumonia and brain damage due to burst blood vessels in the brain. Homeopathic treatment of whooping cough is effective, and especially so if treated early. If the cough continues in spite of well-indicated remedies, allopathic advice should be sought, especially in infants.

TREATMENT

The remedies should be given sparingly, to reduce the chance of aggravation. If aggravation occurs, stop the remedy and wait for improvement to follow. If improvement occurs, stop dosage and repeat only when improvement stops.

■ As a prophylactic to reduce duration and severity, for family and friends.
Pertussin 30c or 200c, one dose per day for 3–5 days.

Early stages

■ Hoarse, dry, choking, convulsive cough, coming on suddenly. Worse at night and by lying down, with anxiety, restlessness and thirst.
Aconite 6c, every 30–60 minutes in the acute stage.

■ Raucous, dry and spasmodic cough, beginning with a runny cold with sneezing, and a watery, nasal discharge irritating the upper lip.
Allium cepa 6c, every 3–4 hours.

■ Dry, noisy, violent, repetitive cough, especially at night, with restlessness, hot, red face, covered with sweat, and bursting feeling in the head. Better from bringing up mucus.
Belladonna 6c, every 1–2 hours.

Established stage

- Spasmodic cough from a constant tickle in the throat, with suffocative spells and blueness of the face, may go quite stiff or bleed from the nose. Wheezing and rattling in the chest, with gagging and vomiting of mucus, but not improved by it.
  Ipecac 6c, every 1–2 hours.

- Dry, frequent, noisy and spasmodic cough, can scarcely breathe between coughs, may retch and gag, cough comes in bouts as if the throat were being tickled. The cough is painful, worse after midnight to around 2 a.m., and better by holding the chest.
  Drosera 6c, every 1–3 hours.

- Violent, explosive, spasmodic cough, cannot be stopped, worse from breathing cold air and followed by profuse vomiting of mucus.
  Corallium rubrum 6c, every 1–2 hours.

- Bouts of coughing bringing up sticky mucus, sometimes with vomiting, worse from 11 p.m. to midnight and in the morning on waking, better from drinking cold water.
  Coccus cacti 6c, every 1–2 hours.

- Spasmodic, dry cough with suffocative bouts and blueness of the face. There may be spasms of the throat and fits of sobbing. The fists may be tightly closed with thumbs tucked in. Symptoms are improved by drinking cold water.
  Cuprum met 6c, every 1–2 hours.

- Cough is mainly dry with little mucus expelled, but is suffocating and blocks expiration.
  Mephitis 6c, every 1–2 hours.

Vaccination

One of the great strides in allopathic medicine has been the considerable increase in life expectancy now enjoyed by the population; but this figure is a matter of statistics. The truth is that a person of 40 now will live only two or three years longer than a person of 40 did in 1900. The apparently greater rise in life expectancy has been achieved by reductions in the infant mortality rate, that is, the chances of survival are now better for babies and young children. This improvement has been attributed to two main factors: the increased standards of hygiene and sanitation now existing in our communities, and vaccination.

There is no question that increased hygiene has contributed to the decreased infantile mortality rate, but this is as much due to increases in general living standards, such as better sewerage and septic tank use, as it is to advances in medicine.

One of the strongest arguments in favor of vaccination is that the chance of complications in infectious diseases is reduced. While vaccination has been of great benefit in underdeveloped countries in controlling infections like polio, diphtheria and measles, and reducing the rate of complication, a deeper problem exists in the bulk of these countries: malnutrition. It is this malnutrition that lowers immune resistance in the first place and sets the stage for the life-threatening complications of infectious diseases common in these countries, especially in the children.

In developed countries the situation is very different, as standards of nutrition and hygiene are much higher. Even so, vaccination is recommended by government. This solution is not a total one, however, as vaccination always has a failure rate (that is, it may not ensure immunity from the disease), which may be 25 per cent or higher. In addition, the incidence of bad reactions to vaccinations is now being examined for the first time, and there is evidence that adverse reactions to vaccinations have been under-reported. So in the end, the advantages vaccination may offer in reducing complications in a disease like measles may be offset by the chance of failure in the vaccination and the possibility of a bad reaction to the vaccine.

The treatment of these infectious disorders by homeopathic medicine is regarded by the profession as largely successful, and the incidence of complications is rare in clinical experience. Furthermore, homeopaths believe that it is important for children to contract these diseases naturally, as it strengthens their immune system and reduces the risk of more serious diseases later in life.

COUNTERING ILL-EFFECTS OF VACCINATION

If you do plan to vaccinate your child, you may also consider using the remedies below to counter any ill-effects and assist in the removal of residual toxins.

- To counter general ill effects. *Vitamin C (calcium ascorbate)* dose according to age, for 1 week before and after vaccination. Mix dose in a little water, fruit juice or cordial. The dose should be reduced if the child complains of digestive discomfort or has loose stools.

Infants up to age 2: 100–250 mg per day.

Children aged 3–5: 250–500 mg per day.

Children over 5: 500 mg–1 g per day.

Homeopathic remedies

- To counter ill effects. *Thuja 30c*, 1 dose per day for 7 days after vaccination.

- To reduce pain, swelling and inflammation. *Arnica 6c*, every 3–4 hours.

GENERAL PROTECTION

If you decide not to vaccinate your child, you need to be aware that you are taking greater responsibility for your child's health, and will need to learn more about medicine. Reading and using this book will help educate you in these areas, as will a regular contact with a local homeopathic practitioner.

The remedies below may be used as a general protection for epidemic diseases whenever they are reported currently in the community. These remedies are not vaccines, and will not prevent the child from getting the illness, as homeopaths believe that it is important for the child to contract the disease naturally and so gain a proper natural immunity. However, the clinical experience of the profession shows that children using these remedies contract the illness in a much milder form, the course of the disease is shortened and the incidence of complications reduced. As a result, the remedies are not true vaccines and are more correctly called prophylactics.

It is important to realize, however, that these remedies have no protective action after the illness has been acquired. Once a child shows a specific illness, such as measles, the remedies in that section should be checked to treat the illness more specifically.

The following remedies are known as nosodes, and are available from homeopathic practitioners. They can be given in any order, but generally only one each month. Initially, give one remedy each month until all have been given: for example, in January give Pertussin, in February give Diptherinum, and so on.

Each year after, you can repeat the process as a booster, but you need to give one dose only of each remedy. Nosodes can also be given as boosters at any time; if you hear of an epidemic of measles in your community, for example, you can give one dose of the measles nosode Morbillinum every day for three days to give your child additional resistance.

TREATMENT

■ Whooping cough.
Pertussin 30c, *once daily for 7 days.*

■ Diptheria.
Diphtherinum 30c, *once daily for 7 days.*

■ Polio.
Polio mix 30c, *once daily for 7 days.*

■ German measles.
Rubella 30c, *once daily for 7 days.*

■ Measles.
Morbillinum 30c, *once daily for 7 days.*

■ Mumps.
Parotidinum 30c, *once daily for 7 days.*

■ Chickenpox.
Varicella 30c, *once daily for 7 days.*

■ Scarlet fever.
Scarlatinum 30c, *once daily for 7 days.*

■ Influenza.
Oscillococcinum 200c, *one dose per day for 7 days.*

■ Glandular fever.
Glandular fever nosode 30c, *once daily for 7 days.*

7

The Treatment
of Mothers

Pregnancy

As we have learned from tragic experience, the fewer drugs a pregnant woman takes the better. Homeopathic remedies carry no such risk of toxicity, and there is no danger of side effects. They are useful in the treatment of many of the minor problems associated with pregnancy, such as backache, incontinence of urine and tired legs. They have considerable value in morning sickness. They have also found good use in the daily work of many midwives, who consider them to be valuable adjuncts to their birth care.

As a preparation

■ Preparation for childbirth, in the third trimester.

Caulophyllum 6c, once daily, or
Caulophyllum 30, once a week.

Cramp in the calves is common during pregnancy and can be very exhausting. It may be due to a mineral deficiency in the mother caused by the nutrient demands of the growing child, so it is important that the mother has a diet with sufficient calcium and magnesium, and adequate salt.

TREATMENT

- The principal remedy when the pain is relieved by pressure, massage and hot applications. *Mag phos 6x, a tissue salt, every 3–4 hours.*

- Cramps with sensation; the parts are asleep, feel numb, cold. *Calc phos 6x, a tissue salt, every 3–4 hours.*

- Cramps with racing mind, tosses at night unable to sleep. *Coffea cruda 6c, every 3–4 hours.*

- Weary feeling in the legs, cramps in the calves and the soles. *Cuprum met 6c, every 3–4 hours.*

- Cramp in the calves and the soles of the feet, with numbness and tingling in the arms and hands, worse by cold. *Nux vomica 6c, every 3–4 hours.*

- Cramp worse in the calves, but relieved by warmth and walking. *Veratrum alb 6c, every 3–4 hours.*

- Cramps mainly in the left leg, better by very hard pressure. *Colocynthis 6c, every 3–4 hours.*

- Legs feel cold and numb, and are better by cold applications. *Ledum 6c, every 3–4 hours.*

CRAVINGS DURING PREGNANCY

Cravings can be viewed without much concern. If the cravings become excessive, the following remedies can be used until they stop.

TREATMENT

- Craving for pickles, vinegar, sour food and drink. *Sepia 6c, every 3–4 hours.*

- Cravings for savory foods. *Pulsatilla 6c, every 3–4 hours.*

- Cravings are unusual and changeable, often seemingly indigestible, but woman feels better for eating them. *Ignatia 6c, every 3–4 hours.*

- Cravings for sweets, sugar, fat and butter.
  Sulphur 6c, every 3–4 hours.
- Craves sugar and sweet foods, has rumbling wind.
  Lycopodium 6c, every 3–4 hours.
- Craves salty foods and extra salt.
  Carbo veg 6c, every 3–4 hours.
- Cravings for chalk.
  Calc carb 6c, every 3–4 hours.
- Cravings for wood or ashes.
  Carbo veg 6c, every 3–4 hours.
- Cravings for dry food, e.g., oatmeal.
  Alumina 6c, every 3–4 hours.

GENITAL HERPES DURING PREGNANCY

Genital herpes in the mother can be passed on to the child, with risk of localisation in the nervous system and the possibility of complications such as meningitis or encephalitis.

Infection can be fatal to babies, so if the herpes virus is active in the mother's birth canal at the time of birth the baby will have to be delivered by cesarean section. As a result, stress during the last weeks of pregnancy should be avoided, and the dietary intake of grains and nuts reduced if there is the chance or a history of herpes. Great care has to be taken with the newborn to avoid passing on the infection through casual contact or kissing.

TREATMENT

- As a general preventative, in susceptible mothers, in the last weeks of pregnancy.
  Herpes progenitalis nosode 30c, 1 dose daily for 1 week.
- As a general treatment, as soon as irritation is suspected.
  Borax 6c, every 3–4 hours.
- Itching lesions forming thick, yellow crusts.
  Petroleum 6c, every 3–4 hours.

MOODS DURING PREGNANCY

The changeable moods during pregnancy are often associated with hormonal changes, and the need for emotional security and reassurance. The following remedies can be used if the moods become marked.

TREATMENT

- Mild, gentle and yielding disposition, changeable moods, sad and crying often, wanting comfort and consolation.
  Pulsatilla 6c, every 3–4 hours.
- Irritable, depressed, fears evil.
  Cimicifuga 6c, every 3–4 hours.
- Irritable and wants to be held, but not improved by it.
  Chamomilla 6c, every 3–4 hours.

- Irritable and wants to be alone, worse by consolation.
  Sepia 6c, every 3–4 hours.
- Depressed, anxious and worried, seeking solitude, worse by consolation.
  Nat mur 6c, every 3–4 hours.
- Fatigue, with yellowness of the face, pigmentation spots on skin and falling hair.
  Sepia 6c, every 3–4 hours.

MORNING SICKNESS

Nausea and vomiting are the most common and distressing disorders of pregnancy. The symptoms usually appear immediately on rising from bed in the morning, and may continue for any length of time during the day. Morning sickness usually continues until about the sixteenth week, but it may also continue for the duration of the pregnancy.

Excessive vomiting in pregnancy should always be viewed cautiously, if for no other reason than it drastically reduces the nourishment of the mother, and can seriously deplete her reserves. The usual treatment is bed rest, and a light, bland and easily digestible diet. In the main, homeopathic medicines are effective treating this condition, especially if given early. Intractable cases require professional advice. Watch for signs of miscarriage.

TREATMENT

- Vomiting often 3–5 p.m., with "gone" feeling. Emptiness in stomach with appetite, but averse to thought of food. Sensitive to smell of partner.
  Sepia 6c, every 3–4 hours.

- Vomiting, nausea worse lying down, but after vomiting feels no better. Profuse saliva, with vomiting of bile or diarrhea.
  Ipecac 6c, every 3–4 hours.

- Inclination to vomit, with sick headache. Great weakness, hollow "gone" feeling. Nausea at the sight, smell or thought of food.
  Cocculus 6c, every 3–4 hours.
- Constant nausea and vomiting in the first trimester. Everything swallowed is vomited, nausea is made worse by eating. Very sensitive, fidgety, restless.
  Asarum 6c, every 3–4 hours.
- Nausea and vomiting worse in the morning, with irritability. Wants to be warm and indoors, very sensitive. May have insomnia and constipation.
  Nux vomica 6c, every 3–4 hours.
- Incessant nausea, day and night, without vomiting.
  Tabacum 6c, every 3–4 hours.
- Faint feeling, as if must eat, but the thought and smell of food disgusts. Eating followed by nausea and vomiting. Dry retching and nausea predominate, often with only saliva and watery fluid being expelled.
  Colchicum 6c, every 3–4 hours.
- Nausea and giddiness, with cold sweat and deathlike pallor, better in fresh cold air. Violent vomiting with cold sweat, on moving.
  Tabacum 6c, every 3–4 hours.
- Vomiting many times each day, with pain, retching and cramps.
  Cuprum acet 6c, every 3–4 hours.
- Nausea and vomiting, with sweat, prostration and shortness of breath. Profuse, watery saliva. Worse from tobacco, slightest motion.
  Lobelia 6c, every 3–4 hours.
- Incessant nausea, with or without vomiting, with accumulation of water in the mouth. Worse from passive motion, from light, noise or attempting to sit up.
  Petroleum 6c, every 3–4 hours.
- Vomiting of any food almost as soon as it is swallowed, with thirst for long, cold drinks.
  Phosphorus 6c, every 3–4 hours.
- Intense but not persistent nausea, with thirst for cold water, little and often, and relief after vomiting.
  Ant tart 6c, every 3–4 hours.
- Nausea throughout pregnancy, but little vomiting. Often worse before midday, avoids the hot sun, and made worse by the heat of the bed.
  Sulphur 6c, every 3–4 hours.
- Vomiting all food throughout whole of pregnancy, leading to exhaustion. Warm water relieves for a while, then nausea returns. Burning belches. Averse to the thought and smell of food.
  Arsenicum 6c, every 3–4 hours.
- Exhaustion after loss of fluids from persistent vomiting.
  China 6c, every 3–4 hours.

- Obstinate cases, with loss of appetite and taste, constant flow of water from mouth.
  Nat mur 6c, a tissue salt, every 3–4 hours.

- Deathly nausea with continuous vomiting, violent retching, worse from motion. When other remedies fail.
  Symphoricarpus racemosa 30c, 1 dose per day.

PHYSICAL PROBLEMS

The physical problems of pregnancy are associated with the structural changes occurring within the body as the baby grows and the mother's body adjusts to the strain. The following remedies can give great relief in the last two months.

TREATMENT

- Backache with sense of weakness and dragging down.
  Kali carb 6c, every 3–4 hours.
- Sore, bruised feeling in abdomen, from pressure of the baby.
  Bellis perennis 6c, every 3–4 hours.
- Backache with lameness, bruised sensation, and difficulty in walking.
  Bellis perennis 6c, alternating with Arnica 6c, every 3–4 hours.
- Hemorrhoids during pregnancy and after birth. Feel bruised and swollen.
  Arnica 6c, every 3–4 hours.
- Hemorrhoids during pregnancy and after birth, with stinging.
  Apis 6c, every 3–4 hours.
- Varicose veins during pregnancy.
  Externally, tincture of Hamamelis 6c, alternating with Pulsatilla 6c, every 3–4 hours.
  Internally, Hamamelis 6c, alternating with Pulsatilla 6c, every 3–4 hours.

- Urine burning and scalding, coming only in drops.
  Cantharis 12c, every 3–4 hours.
- Incontinence of urine, expelled by coughing or sneezing.
  Causticum 6c, every 3–4 hours.
- Constipation, with irritability and frequent ineffectual desire.
  Nux vomica 6c, every 3–4 hours.
- Diarrhea, with violent colic, yellow–greenish stools and irritability.
  Chamomilla 6c, every 3–4 hours.
- Diarrhea, with colic; watery, slimy, greenish stools always different, bitter taste in mouth.
  Pulsatilla 6c, every 3–4 hours.
- Frequent urge to stool or urinate.
  Nux vomica 6c, every 3–4 hours.
- Diarrhea, from cold or getting wet.
  Dulcamara 6c, every 3–4 hours.

Tickling, burning or pricking sensations in the lower legs causing involuntary movement, twitching or jerking are fairly common during pregnancy. The cause is unknown, although it is often associated with a deficiency of iron or vitamin B.

TREATMENT

■ Restlessness caused by stiffness and cramping, must constantly move to seek relief.
Rhus tox 6c, every 3–4 hours.

■ Legs twitching and jerking, with an irresistible urge to move them constantly.
Tarentula 6c, every 3–4 hours.

■ Trembling, twitching and restless legs, even when asleep.
Zincum met 6c, every 3–4 hours.

■ Restlessness from anxiety, with legs constantly moving even though exhausted, worse around midnight.
Arsenicum 6c, every 3–4 hours.

Miscarriage

Miscarriage is the loss of the fetus from the womb before the sixth month; after this time it is called premature labor. Miscarriage can occur at any period of the pregnancy, but most frequently at the third or fourth month. Miscarriage in the first two months is not particularly serious physically, but the flooding that accompanies miscarriage increases as the pregnancy advances. Miscarriages ocurring later than the fourth month are more serious, and often dangerous.

The loss of blood in repeated miscarriage may impair the constitution and lead to more chronic trouble later on, particularly in women already worn down from childbearing and fatigue. Women who miscarry once are likely to miscarry again at about the same time, particularly at the time when the menstrual period would have been due. The use of the homeopathic remedies given here can do much to sustain the pregnancy at these times.

It should be borne in mind that failure of the fetus to thrive is always a possible reason for a miscarriage, and so a miscarriage should not be viewed as totally without purpose in normal body function.

In history of miscarriage

- Tendency to miscarry in the earlier half of pregnancy.
  Sabina 200c, 1 dose per week from the beginning of pregnancy, or 1 dose in the evening for a few days around the time of the previous miscarriage.

- Tendency to abort at the third month, with pains flying across abdomen, forcing to double up.
  Cimificuga 200c, 1 dose per week from the second to the fifth month.

- For women who miscarry easily at about the third month, especially when overtired, with persistent backache and low uterus.
  Kali carb 200c, 1 dose per week from the second to the fifth month.

- Threatened miscarriage around the fifth to seventh month, with chronic heaviness and dragging in the pelvis.
  Sepia 200c, 1 dose per week, starting at about the fourth month.

- For women with delicate and sensitive skin, yellow or brown pigmentation spots, hair falling out and great fatigue. As a constitutional treatment.
  Sepia 200c, 1 dose per week, for a few doses, every 3 months.

- Threatened miscarriage at about the third month, with pains from the small of the back around to the abdomen, ending in crampy, squeezing, bearing-down pressure, tearing down the thighs.
  Viburnum op 200c, 1 dose per week from the second to the fifth month.

- For women of mild, gentle disposition, changeable moods and crying readily, seeking comfort and consolation. As a constitutional treatment.
  Pulsatilla 200c, 1 dose per week for a few weeks, every 3 months.

Threatened miscarriage

The following symptoms generally precede a threatened miscarriage:

- chilliness followed by more or less fever and bearing-down pains
- severe pains in the abdomen, or cutting pains in the loins, resembling labor pains; often the pains come from a point between the spine and the uterus, and come forward to the pubis
- discharge of mucus and blood, sometimes bright red, at other times dark and clotted, followed by a flow of thin, watery blood.

In cases of threatened miscarriage, the patient should immediately lie down, and remain there until the danger has passed. Threatened miscarriage with fever and sweating may indicate a septic condition, and should receive allopathic treatment immediately. The following remedies can be used while allopathic advice is being sought.

- Threatened miscarriage after a shock or fright, with restlessness and thirst, dry skin and great anxiety.
  Aconite 6c, every 30–60 minutes until improved.

- Threatened miscarriage after blow, fall, overexertion, or accident.
  Arnica 6c, every 30 minutes, or Arnica 200c, 1 dose every 4 hours for a few doses.

- Threatened miscarriage from heavy lifting, resulting in dragging pain, tenderness and restlessness, with pressure in the abdomen and some blood.
  Cinnamon 6c, every 30–60 minutes until improved.

- Great pains in the abdomen and loins, with pain in the back as if broken, and bearing down as if the intestines would be pressed out, and a discharge of blood.
  Belladonna 6c, every 30–60 minutes until improved.

- Threatened miscarriage after emotional shock, with hysteria, restlessness and weeping, rapid change of emotions, and irregular, spasmodic uterine pain.
  Ignatia 6c, every 30–60 minutes until improved.

- Severe pain in the back and loins, with a discharge of dark-colored blood.
  Chamomilla 6c, every 15–30 minutes until improved.

- Pains from the small of the back around to the abdomen, ending in crampy, squeezing, bearing-down pressure, tearing down the thighs. Irritable, wants to be alone.
  Viburnum op 6c, every 15–30 minutes until improved.

- Sense of heat and soreness in the womb, especially at the third or fourth month. Pains from small of back to pubis, with cramping and bleeding, worse from any movement.
  Sabina 6c, every 30–60 minutes until improved.

- Threatened miscarriage around the seventh month, with bearing-down sensations and urgent desire for stool, as if all organs would escape.
  Lilium tig 6c, every 30–60 minutes until improved.

- Pains flying across abdomen, forcing to double up, with chills and pricking in the breasts.
  Cimificuga 200c, 1 dose per day for a few days.

- Discharge of dark clotted blood, with a sensation of moving or fluttering in the abdomen, and increased flow of blood on the slightest movement.
  Crocus 6c, every 30 minutes until improved.
- Irregular, feeble, tormenting pains, with scanty or long continued flow, passive oozing, backache, weakness and internal trembling.
  Caulophyllum 6c, every 30–60 minutes until improved.

- Bleeding comes and goes, with spasmodic pains, exciting suffocation or fainting, and craving fresh air.
  Pulsatilla 6c, every 30–60 minutes until improved.
- Severe, forcing, bearing-down pains, with anxiety and debility. Flow of dark blood, with numbness and tingling of extremities.
  Secale 6c, every 30–60 minutes until improved.
- For restoring energy, in exhaustion after loss of blood.
  China 6c, every 3–4 hours.

True miscarriage

If miscarriage does occur, the patient should remain lying, and the appropriate remedies given below can be used while immediate allopathic advice is being sought.

- Acute hemorrhage, with continuous flow of bright red blood, nausea, weakness, pale face, even convulsion without loss of consciousness.
  Ipecac 6c, every 10–15 minutes, until improvement begins.
- Discharge of blood that is partly liquid, partly clotted, with sudden collapse. Gushes of blood, worse from the least motion. Pains from small of back to pubis.
  Sabina 6c, 1 dose every 30 minutes for a few doses. Repeat if necessary.
- Blood light, fluid painless.
  Millefolium 6c, every 15 minutes until improved.

- Persistent hemorrhage.
  Thlapsi 6c, every 15 minutes until improved.
- As a restorative after miscarriage, in women with sensation of weakness, dragging and weight in the pelvis, with sore and tender uterus, great languor and prostration, excessive secretion of saliva.
  Helonias 200c, 1 dose per week for several months.
- For restoring energy, in exhaustion after loss of blood.
  China 200c, 1 dose per day for 3 days.

Labor

Childbirth is a natural process and, unless complications develop, allopathic intervention is seldom needed. A growing number of couples now accept this view, and homeopathic remedies are finding an increasingly useful place in the medicine kits of those who prefer home births and in the dispensaries of midwives. If complications arise, the accompanying remedies should be used while allopathic advice is being sought.

TREATMENT

As a preparation for labor

Labor is usually preceded by pains that commence in the back and run to the loins, or begin in the lower front of the abdomen and run to the back. They may be spaced apart from 30 minutes to several hours.

- For easing of labor, and to improve uterine muscle tone.
  Caulophyllum 30c, 1 dose daily for the last 3 weeks of pregnancy.
- Fetus positioned poorly, in gentle changeable types, seeking comfort.
  Pulsatilla 200c, one dose every 5 days until correction occurs.
- To reduce bruising, bleeding.
  Arnica 200c, 1 dose before labour.

- As a general regulator when labor commences, in the absence of unusual symptoms, and to increase the strength of the contractions.
  Pulsatilla 6c, 1 dose every hour.
- As a preventative against sepsis.
  Pyrogen 30c, 1 dose on commencement of labor, and then every morning for 10 days.

False labor pains

False labor pains differ from true labor pains in that they are irregular, colicky, not increasing in intensity and principally confined to the abdomen. The abdomen is sensitive to pressure and movement.

- False pains, irregular, sharp and colicky, from small of back around to abdomen.
  Cimicifuga 6c, 1 dose per hour for a few hours.

- Irregular, feeble, tormenting pains, with backache, weakness and internal trembling.
  Caulophyllum 6c, 1 dose per hour for a few hours.

To assist labor and shorten its duration

Labor is often protracted and accompanied by considerable distress. The remedies here will do much to shorten the duration and reduce the pain.

■ Pains sharp and rapid, with anxiety, restlessness, fear of death.
Aconite 6c, every 15–30 minutes.

■ Pains in quick succession, ineffectual and violent, with great agitation and tossing about.
Coffea 6c, every 15–30 minutes.

■ Mother seems oversensitive to pain, or suffering out of proportion to pain, restless and greatly anguished. Irritable with pain, cannot bear it.
Chamomilla 6c, every 15–30 minutes.

■ Slow labor in mild, tearful types, with distress and suffocation at each contraction, craving fresh air.
Pulsatilla 6c, 1 dose per hour.

■ Labor protracted, with indefinite pains at long intervals, running to exhaustion.
Caulophyllum 6c, every 30 minutes for a few hours.

■ Stitching pains in the uterus with each contraction, impeding progress, often with backache, weariness and faintness.
Sepia 6c, 1 dose every hour for a few hours.

■ Labor protracted, with irregular and insufficient pains, constant desire to evacuate bladder and rectum.
Nux vomica 6c, every 30 minutes.

■ Strong contraction followed by several weak ones, with no progress, accompanied by headache and numbness in the legs.
Cocculus 6c, 1 dose every 30 minutes.

■ Labor protracted, with intermittent and painless contractions, and intense weariness out of proportion to the suffering.
Gossypium 6c, 1 dose per hour.

■ Contraction is followed by violent pain in lower back, as if it would split open, running down into the hips or buttocks. Often with digestive wind, needing belching to relieve.
Kali carb 6c, 1 dose every 30 minutes.

■ Labor pains attended by spasm of the stomach and vomiting, or with feeble contractions, great fatigue, burning heat and exhaustion.
Secale 6c, 1 dose every 30 minutes.

■ Retained placenta, with pains from sacrum to pubis, or with pains shooting up the vagina.
Sabina 6c, 1 dose per hour.

Preventative care against sepsis

The routine use of homeopathic remedies after labor has led to those obstetricians involved rarely seeing the septic or circulatory complications that are otherwise common.

■ As a preventative against sepis.
  Pyrogen 30c, *1 dose on commencement of labor, and then every morning for 10 days.*

Relief and comfort after labor

■ As an antiseptic application to the vagina after birth, and for pain or tearing.
  Hypericum *and* **calendula** *tinctures combined (***Hypercal***), diluted 1 in 5, and applied locally and renewed daily for 7 days.*

■ After long labor, mother strained and chilled.
  Rhus tox 6c, *every 2–3 hours.*

■ Stretched pains after birth.
  Staphysagria 6c, *every 2–3 hours.*

■ For slicing, stinging pain after laceration or episiotomy.
  Staphysagria 6c, *every time pain returns.*

■ Sharp, shooting pain after laceration or episiotomy.
  Hypericum 6c, *every time pain returns.*

■ For shock and excitement following labor, cannot sleep or pass urine.
  Aconite 6c, *every 3–4 hours.*

■ For relief and comfort afterwards from bruised pain.
  Arnica 200c, *1 dose per day for 3 days.*

■ For violent afterpains.
  Arnica 6c, *every 2–3 hours.*

Post Partum

The use of homeopathic remedies in post-partum treatment has the advantage of being completely non-toxic, and with no ill effects on the baby, the mother, or the milk.

TREATMENT

- No confidence in caring for baby, seems possessed of two wills. Discouraged and untrusting, blames others.
Anacardium 30c, 1 dose a day for 3 days.
- Overwhelmed by depression and gloom, wants never to be pregnant again because of the pain, loss of will to live.
Aurum met 30c, 1 dose a day for 3 days.

- Indifference to husband and children, with desire for solitude.
Sepia 30c, 1 dose a day for 3 days.
- Indifference, with love of sympathy, touch and massage.
Phosphorus 30c, 1 dose a day for 3 days.
- Changeable moods, tearful, seeks company and consolation.
Pulsatilla 30c, 1 dose a day for 3 days.

FLOODING

TREATMENT

- Flooding, with cutting pains around the navel, much nausea and coldness.
Ipecac 6c, every 15–30 minutes.
- Discharge of blood, partly liquid, partly clotted, worse from the least motion. Pains from small of back to pubis.
Sabina 6c, one dose every 30 minutes for a few doses. Repeat if necessary.
- Blood excessive, light, fluid and painless.
Millefolium 6c, every 15 minutes.

- Flooding with pressure in genitals as if everything would fall out, heat in head, and palpitations.
Belladonna 6c, every 15 minutes for a few doses.
- Flooding with dizziness or loss of consciousness, with twitch or convulsion.
China 6c, every 15 minutes for a few doses. See a doctor if China does not resolve.
- Persistent hemorrhage.
Thlapsi 6c, every 15 minutes.

TREATMENT

- Hair loss after childbirth, with premature graying.
  Lycopodium 6c, *every 3–4 hours for 2 weeks, then wait.*
- Hair falls out in handfuls.
  Phosphorus 6c, *every 3–4 hours for 2 weeks, then wait.*

- Hair loss after childbirth, with irritability and indifference to loved ones.
  Sepia 6c, *every 3–4 hours for two weeks, then wait.*

RESTORATION OF ENERGY

TREATMENT

- For restoring energy, in exhaustion after loss of blood.
  China 200c, *1 dose a day for 3 days. It may be repeated every week or so as desired during lactation.*

- Exhaustion with nausea and headache, weak empty feeling, especially after loss of sleep.
  Cocculus 6c, *2 doses a day for a few days.*

Breastfeeding

The problems of breastfeeding center around problems with milk supply, weakness during lactation, and painful breasts and nipples. Homeopathic remedies are of great use here, and rarely fail when well prescribed.

TREATMENT

Local treatment

- As a local application for sore and swollen breasts.
  Fenugreek seeds, powdered in a coffee grinder, mixed with hot water to a thick paste and applied on gauze when warm.

- As a local application, when milk flow is poor.
  Castor oil, *applied on some gauze to the breast when not feeding.*

Milk problems

- Too little milk or milk watery and thin, in mild, tearful types.
  Pulsatilla 6c, every 3–4 hours.
- Milk watery and thin, in fearful types.
  Calc carb 6c, every 3–4 hours.
- Not enough milk, or milk of poor quality.
  Ricinis com 6c, every 3–4 hours.
- Flow too copious.
  Belladonna 6c, every 3–4 hours.

- Milk continues to be secreted after feeding.
  Pulsatilla 6c, every 3–4 hours.
- Loss of milk; breasts decrease in size. Mother thirsty and depressed.
  Lac defloratum 6c, every 3–4 hours.
- Child averse to mother's milk, from poor quality.
  Silicea 6c, a tissue salt, every 3–4 hours.

Painful breasts and nipples

- Nipples burning or smarting after nursing.
  Sulphur 6c, every 3–4 hours.
- Mother weeps when nursing, from the pain.
  Pulsatilla 6c, every 3–4 hours.
- Nipples chap badly.
  Sulphur 6c, every 3–4 hours.
- Cracked, sore nipples, excessively tender. Swelling of the breasts, with violent itching.
  Castor equi 6c, every 3–4 hours.
- Nipple cracks, deep and sore.
  Sepia 6c, every 3–4 hours.
- Nipple cracks across the crown.
  Sepia 6c, every 3–4 hours.
- Nipples drawn in.
  Silicea 6c, a tissue salt, every 3–4 hours.
- Nipples inflamed, extremely tender and sensitive.
  Chamomilla 6c, every 3–4 hours.

- Breasts hot, red, swollen, very painful and tender.
  Belladonna 6c, every 3–4 hours.
- Breasts swollen after weaning, intensely sore.
  Pulsatilla 6c, every 3–4 hours.
- Breasts engorged after weaning, with pain on moving.
  Bryonia 6c, every 3–4 hours.
- Mastitis from blow or injury.
  Arnica 6c, every 3–4 hours.
- Breasts hard and painful, worse from slightest movement.
  Bryonia 6c, every 3–4 hours.
- Pain in nipple while nursing.
  Phellandrium 6c, every 3–4 hours.
- Sharp pain in breast while nursing.
  Silicea 6c, a tissue salt, every 3–4 hours.
- Pain shoots through to shoulder blade while nursing.
  Croton tig 6c, every 3–4 hours.

- Abscess, with pain and hardness, worse with movement.
  Bryonia 6c, every 3–4 hours.
- Suppuration from the nipple, with burning, watery, offensive discharge.
  Phosphorus 6c, every 3–4 hours.
- Breasts swollen, hard and thickened, nipples sore, cracked and blistered.
  Graphites 6c, every 3–4 hours.
- Breasts red, throbbing and heavy, worse from lying down.
  Belladonna 6c, every 3–4 hours.

- Breasts large and painful because of fluid retention.
  Nat mur 6x, a tissue salt, every 3–4 hours.
- Enlargement with pain and tenderness.
  Conium 6c, every 3–4 hours.
- Enlarged breasts with darting pains.
  Carbo animalis 6c, every 3–4 hours.

Weakness during breastfeeding

- Weakness from loss of vital fluids, during delivery and from breastfeeding. Lethargic, with poor digestion.
  China 6c, every 3–4 hours.

- Weakness, loss of weight, no energy, susceptible to cold, with pain in the back during breastfeeding.
  Silicea 6x, a tissue salt, every 3–4 hours.

8

The Treatment of Women

Absent Periods

Lessening of the menstrual flow may occur in varying degrees. It may accompany anorexia, extreme weight loss and excessive exercise. It most commonly comes on suddenly, often after emotional shock, exposure to cold or damp weather, or getting the feet wet and cold close to menstruation. In rare cases, it may be due to a displacement of the uterus, although this can often be corrected by special exercises.

TREATMENT

■ Suppression of flow with depressed spirits, lassitude and debility. Constant dull headache, fidgety, cross and irritable.
Ferrum phos 6x, a tissue salt, 3 times a day for 1 month.

■ Periods absent in nervy, chilly, tired, overweight women. Breasts swollen and painful, legs heavy.
Calc carb 6c, 3 times a day for 1 month.

■ Scanty or suppressed periods, with weight and fullness of the abdomen.
Kali sulph 6x, a tissue salt, 3 times a day for 1 month.

■ Periods stop suddenly due to emotional shock or exposure to dry cold.
Aconite 6c, 3 times a day for 1 month.

- No periods in anemic types.
  Calc phos 6x, a tissue salt, 3 times a day for 1 month.
- In young girls when menses do not appear, or when scanty and at long intervals.
  Nat mur 6x, a tissue salt, 3 times a day for 1 month.
- Periods stop from chill after exercise.
  Dulcamara 6c, 3 times a day for 1 month.
- Periods stop after grief or shock.
  Ignatia 6c, 3 times a day for 1 month.

- Periods absent, with headaches, constipation, irritability.
  Nat mur 6x, a tissue salt, 3 times a day for 1 month.
- Periods absent, with tearfulness and irritability, loss of sex drive and fear of losing control.
  Sepia 6c, 3 times a day for 1 month.
- Weakness and weariness, face pale but flushes easily, wants to sit down often.
  Ferrum met 6c, 3 times a day for 1 month.

Breast Lumps and Congestion

Any lump should receive professional assessment, but particularly any that are generally painless, more or less constant in size, and especially if the nipple is drawn in. Cancer especially requires allopathic advice.

Homeopathic remedies cannot treat all the minor disorders of breasts, and if there is no clear-cut improvement after 1–2 months professional advice should be sought. But there are a number of remedies that have a selective action on the breasts, and are particularly useful in premenstrual congestion there, and in the case of benign tumors.

TREATMENT

- Premenstrual congestion of the breasts, during the whole or second part of the menstrual cycle.
  Lac caninum 12c, morning and evening from day 14 to the start of the next period.

- Premenstrual congestion of the breasts, pain worse from the slightest movement.
  Bryonia 12c, every 3–4 hours.
- Premenstrual congestion in women with very large breasts.
  Calc carb 6c, every 3–4 hours.
- Premenstrual breast congestion in women with abundant periods, weight gain and nervousness before the period.
  Folliculinum 9c, 1 dose on day 7 of the cycle, and 1 dose on day 21.
- Cyst in the breast, hard and painful but itchy, with stitching pains in the nipple. Discomfort worse just before and after the period; woman wants to press breasts hard with hand.
  Conium 6c, 2 doses a day for several months.
- Bluish-red lumps in the breast, with gradual loss of fatty tissue, and tendency to feel hot all the time.
  Iodum 6c, every 3–4 hours.
- Cyst in the breast, with purplish tinge to the tissue, tender before and during the period. Worse from chill, damp weather and emotional strain.
  Phytolacca 6c, 2 doses a day for several months.
- Firm lumps of the breast with pain before or during the periods.
  Phytolacca 12c, 2 doses a day for several months.
- Breast lumps after a blow.
  Conium 6c, 2 doses a day for several months.

Delayed Periods

The menstrual cycle is longer in some women than others, and a longer or shorter cycle should not be viewed as cause for concern. Delayed periods may occur from emotional upset, pregnancy, as an after-effect of the contraceptive pill and during the onset of menopause.

TREATMENT

- Periods absent after fright or sudden exposure to cold.
  Aconite 6c, every 3–4 hours.
- Periods absent after fright, with changeable moods.
  Pulsatilla 6c, every 3–4 hours.
- Periods absent after weaning.
  Sepia 6c, every 3–4 hours.
- Periods delayed, with hot, flushing skin, faintness in the late morning.
  Sulphur 6c, every 3–4 hours.

Heavy Periods and Flooding

Heavy bleeding should always be viewed with caution, for even if painless can be due to a variety of underlying disorders, including fibroids, polyps, cysts, tumors and hormonal imbalance. Failure to respond to homeopathic medicines indicates the need for professional treatment.

TREATMENT

- Periods too frequent and too profuse and painful, with congestion and bright-red blood.
  Ferrum phos 6x, a tissue salt, every 3–4 hours.

- Periods intermittent, with cramping and faintness, passing dark clots.
  China 6c, every 3–4 hours.

- Periods too early, heavy and prolonged, may gush on each movement, with sharp pains from the back to abdomen or upwards from the vagina.
  Sabina 6c, every 3–4 hours.

- Periods are heavy and prolonged, coming on every 15 days, with pain in the lower back and a tendency to faint.
  Trillium 6c, every 3–4 hours.

- Painful cramps, with throbbing, dragging pains and hot, bright-red blood.
  Belladonna 6c, every 3–4 hours.

- Flooding with clots of blackish blood, sensation of movement in the abdomen.
  Crocus 6c, every 3–4 hours.

- Periods too early and lasting too long, with irritability.
  Nux vomica 6c, every 3–4 hours.

- Periods irregular and profuse, with bloating, moodiness and irritability.
  Sepia 6c, every 3–4 hours.

- Periods profuse, with dark clotted blood, almost black.
  Kali mur 6x, a tissue salt, every 3–4 hours.

- Profuse periods with bearing-down pains.
  Calc fluor 6x, a tissue salt, every 3–4 hours.

- Profuse bleeding with nausea, cramps down into the thighs, worse during the first few days of the period and at night. Muffled buzzing in the ears.
  Borax 6c, every 3–4 hours.

- Periods profuse and changeable, no two alike, with intermittent bleeding.
  Pulsatilla 6c, every 3–4 hours.

- Periods profuse, with cramping pains, must cross legs.
  Sepia 6c, every 3–4 hours.

- Periods painless and heavy, with exhaustion.
  China 6c, every 3–4 hours.
- Heavy periods with nausea and bright-red blood. Bright-red blood breaking through between periods.
  Ipecac 6c, every 3–4 hours.
- Flooding with dark and watery blood, face pale, occasional flushing, better from gentle movement.
  Ferrum 6c, every 3–4 hours.

Menopause

Menopausal problems are commonly associated with hormonal imbalance. They include flushing, irregular periods, flooding and emotional instability. A great many women endure upsetting symptoms of menopause, believing that nothing can be done. Homeopathic medicines have achieved many dramatic cures here. Dosage is generally the 6c potency for 2 weeks, but professional advice should be sought in resistant cases.

TREATMENT

- Hot flashes with red face, alternating with pale face.
  Ferrum phos 6x, a tissue salt, every 3–4 hours.
- Flushing in to the head and face, starting and stopping suddenly, with sweat, redness, throbbing and congestion.
  Belladonna 6c, morning and evening.
- Hot flushing in the face and neck, with circular redness of the cheeks and burning in the ears.
  Sanguinaria 6c, every 3–4 hours.
- Hot flashes with redness, congestion, and pounding heart.
  Glonoine 6c, morning and evening.
- Flashes of heat, with flooding, irritability, hysteria, and rejection of loved ones.
  Sepia 6c, morning and evening.
- Changeable periods and moods, with tearful episodes, seeking comfort and consolation, preferring the open air.
  Pulsatilla 6c, morning and evening.
- Hot flashes with palpitations, loss of appetite, backache, feelings of tautness and nervousness, worse around 3 a.m.
  Kali carb 6c, morning and evening.

- Flashes of heat, always worse after sleep, person very talkative, with strong and fixed ideas.
  Lachesis 12c, morning and evening.
- Flushes especially on the face, with nosebleeds, weight gain, scanty periods, cutting pains in the lower abdomen.
  Graphites 6c, morning and evening.
- Hot flashes coming on suddenly.
  Amyl nit 6c, morning and evening.
- Hot flashes worse in evening and after exercise, great weariness.
  Sulph ac 6c, morning and evening.
- Hot flashes with nervousness, mental depression, irritability, anxiety, fainting spells.
  Kali phos 6x, a tissue salt, every 3–4 hours.
- Dryness and thinning of the walls of the vagina, constipation with burned or blackish-looking stools.
  Bryonia 6c, morning and evening.
- Hot flashes with nervousness, palpitations and tendency to cramps.
  Mag phos 6x, a tissue salt, every 3–4 hours.
- Hot flashes with weak, run-down condition, anemia, loss of weight.
  Calc phos 6x, a tissue salt, every 3–4 hours.

Ovarian Cysts

Cysts are fluid-filled tissues that can develop anywhere. When they occur on the ovaries they often show no symptoms unless they are large enough to press on the bladder, give pain on intercourse, or cause visible swelling in the lower abdomen. Menstrual bleeding may be altered if production of ovarian hormones is affected, and sometimes the menstrual cycle can be irregular. If there is sudden, severe abdominal pain with fever and nausea, the cysts may have burst: seek *urgent allopathic treatment*.

TREATMENT

- Left ovary affected, local pain that is worse in the morning but wears off during the period.
  Lachesis 12c, every 3–4 hours.
- Pain in the lower abdomen, like a wedge being driven through the ovary and uterus.
  Iodum 6c, every 3–4 hours.

- Sore, stinging pains in the right
  ovary, with painful periods and
  local tenderness.
  Apis 6c, every 3–4 hours.

- Pains seeming to bore through
  the lower abdomen, forcing to
  bend double and to press fists
  into abdomen for relief.
  Colocynth 6c, every 3–4 hours.

Period Pain

In spite of its widespread occurrence, period pain is not normal, and
rarely need be endured. The pain can occur before, during or after the
onset of the period, and may be accompanied by headache, irritability
and depression. The pain can take a number of forms, including cramping,
shooting and pressing. The following remedies can be taken for a few
days before the period, and if pain persists.

TREATMENT

- Cramping, labor-like, bearing-
  down pains, coming in spasms.
  Sharp and cutting pains, relieved
  by heat and pressure. Membranes
  sometimes present in the flow.
  *Mag phos 6x, a tissue salt, every
  3–4 hours. Often the only remedy
  needed.*

- Strong contractions of the uterus
  like labor pains, with headaches
  for a few days before the flow.
  Cimicifuga 6c, every 3–4 hours.

- Pain extends down into the
  thighs, with nausea and muffled
  buzzing in the ears.
  Borax 6c, every 3–4 hours.

- Sudden severe pain, with anxiety
  and restlessness.
  Aconite 6c, every 3–4 hours.

- Cutting, dragging pains just
  before the period, with profuse
  bright-red blood, worse from
  lying down, better by moving
  about.
  Belladonna 6c, every 3–4 hours.

- Painful menstruation with
  bright-red flow, flushed face and
  quickened pulse. Vomiting of
  undigested food. Congestion of
  the pelvic organs. Abdomen feels
  full and heavy, beginning several
  days before the flow.
  *Ferrum phos 6x, a tissue salt, every
  3–4 hours. Often taken in alternation
  with Mag phos.*

- Patient intolerant of pain—cannot bear it. Pains often down the thighs, with brown blood.
  Chamomilla 6c, every 3–4 hours.
- Painful menstruation with great restlessness, tossing around in all directions. Tearful, and woman always feels better in open air.
  Pulsatilla 6c, every 3–4 hours.
- Menstrual colic in pale, tearful, irritable, sensitive women, with weakness of the nervous system. Flow deep, dark red.
  Kali phos 6x, a tissue salt, every 3–4 hours.
- Periods painful and changeable, no two the same.
  Pulsatilla 6c, every 3–4 hours.
- Sensation of bearing down and heaviness in pelvic region, dragging pains from sacrum. Great irritability.
  Sepia 6c, every 3–4 hours.
- Spotting between periods. Periods too early, light, but last too long.
  Phosphorus 6c, every 3–4 hours.
- In anemic girls, at puberty, with scanty flow.
  Calc phos 6x, a tissue salt, every 3–4 hours.
- Period pain after taking cold, blood dark or blackish-red.
  Kali mur 6x, a tissue salt, every 3–4 hours.
- Periods late and shorter than usual, with weepiness.
  Pulsatilla 6c, every 3–4 hours.
- Pains labor-like, can be sharp and constricting, extending into the back, and soothed by heat.
  Gelsemium 6c, every 3–4 hours.
- Pains run down the thighs.
  Chamomilla 6c, every 3–4 hours.
- Pains worse on any movement, must lie still and hold abdomen.
  Bryonia 6c, every 3–4 hours.
- Periods late and scanty, often with membranes. The pain begins in the back, goes around to the uterus, ends up in cramps there, may spread to the thighs. Tendency to faint.
  Viburnum 6c, every 3–4 hours.
- Prolonged periods that arrive early, with chilliness, constipation, exhaustion and irritability.
  Nux vomica 6c, every 3–4 hours.
- Heavy, pressing-down feeling, with severe pain in the back, down the thighs and through the hips.
  Cimicifuga 6c, every 3–4 hours.
- Pain from back to pubic bone. Blood is dark, clots easily.
  Sabina 6c, every 3–4 hours.
- Great weakness and languor with melancholia, dragging and weight in sacrum and pelvis.
  Helonias 6c, every 3–4 hours.

- Flow is irritating, dark and scanty, with mental depression. Back pains, relieved by lying on back. Often with throbbing headache and soreness of the eyes.
  Nat mur 6x, a tissue salt, every 3–4 hours.

- Icy coldness of the whole body before and during the flow, with constipation and sweating of the feet.
  Silicea 6x, a tissue salt, every 3–4 hours.

Period Problems in Adolescents

The appearance of menstruation varies, from ages 9 to 18, but is most common between the ages of 12 and 14. In adolescence the treatment of period problems is usually fast and effective. The most common problems are delayed onset, mood changes, heavy or irregular periods, period pain, headaches, and dizziness.

TREATMENT

- First period delayed, in adolescent girls.
  Pulsatilla 6c, morning and evening for several months.

- Periods too early and excessive, with headache.
  Calc phos 6x, a tissue salt, morning and evening for several months.

- Periods in the daytime only.
  Pulsatilla 6c, morning and evening for several months.

- Periods irregular, with bloating, moodiness, and irritability.
  Sepia 6c, morning and evening for several months.

- Periods changeable, no two alike.
  Pulsatilla 6c, morning and evening for several months.

- Periods absent, with bleeding from nose instead.
  Phosphorus 6c, morning and evening for several months.

- Periods with intermittent bleeding; stops and starts.
  Pulsatilla 6c, morning and evening for several months.

- Periods too early in young girls, with flooding.
  Calc phos 6x, a tissue salt, morning and evening for several months.

Premenstrual Tension

Premenstrual tension is often signalled by appetite cravings, tenderness of the breasts, bloating and tenderness of the abdomen, fluid retention, and mood changes such as irritability or tearfulness. Often nutritional deficiency is involved, particularly of vitamin B^6 and essential fatty acids. Hormonal imbalances are commonly a cause. Evening primrose oil is often useful as a supplement.

TREATMENT

- Premenstrual tension in women with abundant periods, breasts feel full, hot, heavy, tense or painful, with weight gain and nervousness before the period.
  Folliculinum 9c, 1 dose on day 7 of the cycle and 1 dose on day 21.

- Tender breasts, fatigue, irritability, senstivity to odors, loss of sex drive and bearing-down sensations with the flow.
  Sepia 6c, every 3–4 hours.

- With angry outbursts and rejection of those most loved.
  Sepia 6c, every 3–4 hours.

- Tearful and changeable, craves company and consolation, always feels better outdoors.
  Pulsatilla 6c, every 3–4 hours.

- Moody, depressed and irritable, seeking solitude, with strong cravings.
  Nat mur 6x, a tissue salt, every 3–4 hours.

- Intense irritability that is worse in morning, with craving for sweet or fatty foods, constipation.
  Nux vomica 6c, every 3–4 hours.

Scanty Periods

Light periods are not necessarily a disorder, and may come at times of change, such as during adolescence, in a time of general ill health, at the onset of menopause, after using the contraceptive pill and after pregnancy. In most cases the flow will re-establish itself without intervention. In cases where the patient feels unwell, the following remedies are of great use.

TREATMENT

- Much lighter after chill, emotional distress, or shock.
  Aconite 6c, *every 3–4 hours.*
- Periods generally light but changeable, in gentle, tearful types.
  Pulsatilla 6c, *every 3–4 hours.*
- Periods too late, scanty, and last too long.
  Pulsatilla 6c, *every 3–4 hours.*
- Light and spotty, in thin, artistic, sensitive women.
  Phosphorus 6c, *every 3–4 hours.*
- Watery periods, in depressed, worrying types who seek solitude.
  Nat mur 6c, *every 3–4 hours.*
- With bearing-down pains, irritability and desire for solitude.
  Sepia 6c, *every 3–4 hours.*

Uterine Fibroids

Fibroids are nonmalignant growths in or on the uterus, especially common in women aged 35–40. They vary in size from a pea to a small apple. They may take years to develop and tend to occur a few at a time. Small fibroids often show no symptoms, but large ones can give rise to heavy periods, painful intercourse, infertility and increases in urinary frequency. The cause is unknown, although estrogens in oral contraceptives may encourage them. Troublesome fibroids must be removed surgically, although homeopathic remedies have produced some remarkable cures. Severe hemorrhage should receive allopathic attention.

TREATMENT

- Fibroids with short periods as menopause approaches, great pain eased by scanty flow, abdomen sensitive to tight clothing.
  Lachesis 12c, *every 4 hours.*
- Menstrual flow heavier than usual, body feels icy cold, with bleeding between periods.
  Silicea 6x, *a tissue salt*, *every 3–4 hours.*

- Uterus feels swollen and painful, with spasmodic contractions of the vagina.
  Aurum mur 6c, *every 3–4 hours.*
- Firm or hard fibroids in older women, often with nodular breasts and a history of celibacy.
  Conium 6c, *every 3–4 hours.*
- Fibroids with a tendency to hemorrhage.
  Phosphorus 6c, *every 3–4 hours.*
- Small fibroids, with profuse, yellow discharge.
  Calc iod 6c, *every 3–4 hours.*

- Fibroids of an elastic consistency.
  Lapis albus 6c, *every 3–4 hours.*
- Continuous bleeding.
  Thlapsi 6c, *every 3–4 hours.*
- Uterus feels as if it is being squeezed during periods.
  Kali iod 6c, *every 3–4 hours.*
- Swollen uterus, with urge to bear down and watery, brown discharge from the vagina between the periods. Painful cramps during the periods.
  Fraxinus 6c, *every 3–4 hours.*

Uterine Prolapse

Prolapse occurs when the ligaments and muscles that hold the uterus in place become weak or stretch, allowing the uterus to protrude into the vagina or press on the bladder or rectum. This can cause a heavy pressure in the abdomen, incontinence or urinary difficulty, and discomfort when passing stool. If symptoms are not too severe, the remedies below will benefit in the first month. If symptoms persist, seek professional advice.

TREATMENT

- Downward pressure in lower abdomen and back pain; tearful types, with nausea and heat. Worse from menstruation.
  Pulsatilla 6c, *every 3–4 hours.*
- Spasms of pain downwards, with irritability and constant urge to pass urine or stool.
  Nux vomica 6c, *every 3–4 hours.*

- Heaviness and dragging in the lower abdomen, worse by bending or lifting and before period, when it feels as if woman must sit down to contain the parts. Depression, irritability and pain on intercourse.
  Sepia 6c, *every 3–4 hours.*

- Pain in lower back; heavy feeling in abdomen and just below ribs, as if abdomen and contents will drop out. Vagina hot, dry. *Belladonna 6c*, *every 3–4 hours.*
- Stretching and pulling sensations in lower abdomen, with heaviness. *Calc fluor*, *a tissue salt, every 3–4 hours.*

- Pain and tenderness in lower abdomen, with nervousness and irritability. Urgent desire to pass urine and stool; vulva itchy, feels as if external support is needed. Better by rest. *Lilium 6c*, *every 3–4 hours.*

Vaginal Discharge

Unusual vaginal discharge is otherwise known as leucorrhea. It is the secretion of an abnormal quantity of mucus from the mucous membrane that lines the vagina and uterus. This mucus may vary in color from a thin, clear fluid to a thick, white or yellow discharge, and may sometimes be tinged with blood. Causes vary, from hormonal imbalances in adolescents, women after childbirth, and older women after menopause, to nervous strain and local infection.

TREATMENT

Wear cotton underwear, changing it daily. Avoid vaginal deodorants, perfumed bath salts and talcum powder. Douche twice daily with 250 ml of warm water to which a teaspoon of tea tree oil has been added. At night apply yogurt on a tampon before retiring. Remedies below should be taken for 1 month.

- Watery, scalding, irritating discharge, smarting after or between the periods. *Nat mur 6x*, *a tissue salt, every 3–4 hours.*
- Discharge clear and very irritating, with scalded feeling on the inside of the thighs. *Borax 6c*, *every 3–4 hours.*

- Discharge of albuminous mucus, like the white of an egg, worse after menstruation. *Calc phos 6x*, *a tissue salt, every 3–4 hours.*
- Discharge of milky-white mucus, non-irritating and profuse. *Kali mur 6x*, *a tissue salt, every 3–4 hours.*

- Watery, cloudy discharge, causing smarting and soreness, worse before and after periods, and when lying down.
  Pulsatilla 6c, every 3–4 hours.
- Itchy, milky discharge, smelling like rye bread, preceded by great weakness, flushed face and pains in the small of the back.
  Kreosotum 6c, every 3–4 hours.
- Milky discharge, causing itching that is worse after passing urine and before menstruation.
  Calc carb 6c, every 3–4 hours.
- Copious, straw-colored discharge, itching and smarting. Itching relieved by cold water.
  Alumina 6c, every 3–4 hours.
- Yellowish, smarting discharge, sharp and itching, with distended abdomen, that is worse during the day.
  Sepia 6c, every 3–4 hours.
- Discharge creamy or honey-colored, acrid and sour-smelling.
  Nat phos 6x, a tissue salt, every 3–4 hours.
- Scalding, acrid discharge, yellow and irritating.
  Kali phos 6x, a tissue salt, every 3–4 hours.
- Greenish discharge that smarts and stings, from suspected *Trichomonas* infection.
  Bovista 6c, every 3–4 hours.
- Stinging discharge with foul smell, containing some solid matter, woman feels chilly and sweaty by turns, from suspected *Trichomonas* infection.
  Mercurius 6c, every 3–4 hours.
- Stringy mucus that is greenish and pinkish, more copious after the period, from suspected *Trichomonas* infection.
  Nitric acid 6c, every 3–4 hours.
- Corrosive greenish discharge, especially before the period, from suspected *Trichomonas* infection.
  Carbo veg 6c, every 3–4 hours.
- White or yellowish discharge that burns and stings, with cramping pains in the abdomen and pinching pains around the navel, worse before the period.
  Sulphur 6c, every 3–4 hours.
- Discharge of yellow or greenish secretion, watery or slimy.
  Kali sulph 6x, a tissue salt, every 3–4 hours.

Vaginal Itching

Itching of the vagina and the external vulva can be intense and distressing. It can be due to skin problems, hormonal imbalances, the use of tampons, irritants in hygienic products, lack of vitamin B in the diet or poor hygiene.

TREATMENT

- Itch with sweaty and smelly groin, worse by heat and washing.
  Sulphur 6c, every 3–4 hours.
- Creeping sensation in vagina that is worse on moving and at night, sex drive increased.
  Caladium 6c, every 3–4 hours.
- Itching with labia swollen and local veins distended.
  Carbo veg 6c, every 3–4 hours.

- Skin very red, with itching relieved by heat.
  Rhus tox 6c, every 3–4 hours.
- Itching aggravated by frequent sex or suppressed desire.
  Conium 6c, every 3–4 hours.
- Itching worse before and after period in overweight women, chilly and sweaty.
  Calc carb 6c, every 3–4 hours.
- Itching worse in the morning, soothed by hot baths and by moving around in the open air.
  Radium brom 6c, every 3–4 hours.

9
The Treatment
of Men

Gout

Although not entirely a male disorder, gout has a tendency to be hereditary and afflict men more than women. Gout is more common in mature
age, and in those who lead a sedentary life with indulgence in rich food
and liquor. In a typical attack there is a severe pain in a joint, usually
the big toe. The joint swells and becomes hot, and any jarring causes
intense pain. In chronic gout the joint becomes permanently enlarged,
and remains tender and sensitive at all times. The diet must be changed
to eliminate foods rich in purines, which include liver, sardines, oysters
and anchovies. The following remedies may be used during acute attacks.

TREATMENT

■ Acute attacks, with fever,
inflammation and pain.
Ferrum phos **6x**, *a tissue salt, every
3–4 hours.*

■ Gout with swollen, red joints
and pains that move from joint
to joint.
Pulsatilla **6c**, *every 3–4 hours.*

- Affected joint hot, red, swollen and stiff, excruciatingly painful, with shooting and tearing pains, especially at night or on moving. Cannot bear even slightest touch.
Colchicum 6c, *every 3–4 hours.*
- Gout with strong-smelling urine.
Benzoic acid 6c, *every 3–4 hours.*
- Gout due to over-indulgence in rich foods, or where bilious symptoms predominate. The tongue has a green–gray coating at the back, or may be clear.
Nat sulph 6x, *a tissue salt, every 3–4 hours.*
- Gout with one foot hot, the other cold, and worse 4–8 p.m.
Lycopodium 6c, *every 3–4 hours.*
- Joints are swollen, purple and puffy, but cold, and improved by cold applications.
Ledum 6c, *every 3–4 hours.*
- In chronic gout, with sour sweat and a creamy tongue at the back.
Nat phos 6x, *a tissue salt, every 3–4 hours.*
- Gout with joints which itch and burn.
Urtica 6c, *every 3–4 hours.*

Hair Loss

Hair loss is sometimes caused by nutritional deficiency, particularly by a lack of zinc, B vitamins and silica in the diet, but is more often caused by many factors combined. Chief amongst these is genetic inheritance, as baldness tends to run in families. Stress also accelerates hair loss, due to constriction of the blood vessels in the scalp which feed the hair follicles; relaxation and daily scalp massage can do much here to slow down the hair loss. Homeopathic treatment is generally constitutional, but the following remedies taken for several weeks and then repeated periodically have had some clinical effect in slowing hair loss. Success should be followed by deeper homeopathic treatment.

TREATMENT

- Falling out of hair, with bald spots. Much scaling of the scalp, moist and sticky. Dandruff.
Kali sulph 6x, *a tissue salt, every 3–4 hours.*
- Hair is brittle and falls out in small tufts.
Fluoric ac 6c, *every 3–4 hours.*

- Impoverished condition of the hair, with a notable lack of luster.
  Silicea 6x, a tissue salt, every 3—4 hours.
- Hair loss with boils on scalp, headaches that worsen at night.
  Aurum met 6c, every 3—4 hours.
- Loss of hair over body as well as the scalp, scalp feels painful when touched.
  Selenium 6c, every 3—4 hours.
- Loss of hair from nervous stress and exhaustion.
  Kali phos 6x, a tissue salt, every 3—4 hours.
- Hair loss and greasy hair after grief or exhaustion, often going gray, with apathy and indifference.
  Phos ac 6c, every 3—4 hours for several weeks.
- Hair loss with dryness of the hair and scalp.
  Kali carb 6c, every 3—4 hours for several weeks.
- Hair loss with dandruff, especially greasy at hairline.
  Nat mur 6x, a tissue salt, every 3—4 hours for several weeks.
- Loss of hair after severe injury.
  Arnica 6c, every 3—4 hours for several weeks.
- Hair falls out in handfuls.
  Phosphorus 6c, every 3—4 hours for several weeks.
- Hair loss due to bad nutrition.
  Calc phos 6x, a tissue salt, every 3—4 hours for several weeks.
- Hair loss with premature baldness and graying, often with eczema behind the ears.
  Lycopodium 6c, every 3—4 hours for several weeks.

Impotence

Impotence is the partial or complete inability for a man to achieve an erection, have intercourse or reach orgasm. It is a complex condition, and most often has a psychological component. Stress is commonly involved, along with fatigue, performance anxiety, identity problems and depression. Treatment involves avoidance of alcohol and stimulants, reducing stress, and being able to relax in a sympathetic, undemanding environment. It is important that once improvement occurs, frequency of intercourse is not increased to excessive levels.

- Lost desire, poor erections, after stress, overwork, illness or excessive intercourse, with apathy.
  Phos ac 6c, morning and evening.
- Loss of sex drive or aversion to sex, with ejaculation premature or absent.
  Graphites 6c, morning and evening.
- Anxiety about intercourse with lack of confidence and fear of failure. Erections poor, even though desire is high. Premature ejaculation may occur.
  Lycopodium 6c, morning and evening.
- Failure to achieve erection or premature ejaculation, from overuse of stimulants in stressed persons, easily irritable.
  Nux vomica 6c, morning and evening.
- Erections poor with general weakness, especially if intercourse has been very frequent.
  Agnus castus 6c, morning and evening.
- Poor erections after frequent intercourse or debilitating weakness.
  China 6c, morning and evening.

- Poor erections even though desire is high, loses semen during sleep.
  Selenium 6c, morning and evening.
- Intense desire but poor erections, often after long periods of abstinence.
  Conium 6c, morning and evening.
- Strong desire but erection is lost. Erections while asleep, but disappear on waking.
  Caladium 6c, morning and evening.
- Loss of potency, with shrunken testes and enlarged prostate.
  Iodum 6c, morning and evening.
- Impotence through failure of erection on penetration, or through lack of desire for sex.
  Arg nit 6c, morning and evening.
- Premature impotence with easy exhaustion and enlarged glands. Looks old before his years.
  Baryta carb 6c, morning and evening.
- Difficulties caused by grief or disappointment in a previous relationship.
  Ignatia 6c, morning and evening.

Prostate Enlargement

The prostate gland lies at the neck of the bladder, and surrounds part of the urethra, which carries the urine from the bladder. Enlargement of the prostate is common in men over 45, and results in a weak stream of urine, incomplete emptying of the bladder and the need for frequent urination at night. Although surgery is commonly recommended, homeopathic remedies have had some excellent results. Coffee and alcohol should be avoided, and an active lifestyle encouraged. Drink 6–8 glasses of water per day.

TREATMENT

- Acute prostatic congestion, with retention of urine, or difficult urination.
  Ferrum phos 6x, a tissue salt, every 3–4 hours.
- Constant desire to pass urine, which is difficult to start and passed only in small quantities. Sharp pains when urinating running from the bladder to the end of the urethra, frequent urge to urinate at night. May be able to pass urine only when standing with legs wide apart and body bending forward.
  Chimaphilla 6c, every 3–4 hours.
- Urination is intermittent, must wait a long time before urine finally passes, and stream is weak. May come initially in drops with burning pain, then flows freely and more painlessly, with dribbling after.
  Clematis 6c, every 3–4 hours.
- Frequent urgent desire to pass urine with burning or cutting sensation at the neck of the bladder.
  Thuja 6c, every 3–4 hours.

- Intermittent stream, with difficulty in completely evacuating the bladder, especially in those affected by excessive intercourse or long abstinence.
  Conium 6c, every 3–4 hours.
- Frequent urge to urinate, with difficult or painful urination, and spasms of the bladder or urethra.
  Sabal 6c, every 3–4 hours.
- Pains on passing urine and at the end of urination, with a heavy sensation in the bladder, not helped by urination.
  Equisetum 6c, every 3–4 hours.
- Prostate enlargement with yellow, turbid urine. Flow is changeable, sometimes free and sometimes restricted.
  Pulsatilla 6c, every 3–4 hours.
- Urination drop by drop, with pain from the kidneys down to the thighs.
  Pareira brav 6c, every 3–4 hours.
- Frequent urination at night, with smarting of the neck of the bladder and pressure on the rectum.
  Ferrum pic 6c, every 3–4 hours.

- Enlargement of the prostate with urging to urinate, but urine is painful.
  Populus trem 6c, every 3–4 hours.

- Enlargement of the prostate, stony hard.
  Calc fluor 6x, a tissue salt, every 3–4 hours.
- Loss of potency, with hard prostate and shrunken testes.
  Iodum 6c, every 3–4 hours.

Stress and Nervous Tension

Although women suffer from stress as well as men, men are currently more likely to suffer from it.

TREATMENT

- Nervous system overactive due to overwork: person finds it hard to let go and relax, even in bed.
  Tarentula 6c, every 3–4 hours.
- Oversensitive to many influences, with anxiety, repeated sighing, insomnia, palpitations, loss of appetite, better when the mind is occupied. Often after emotional shock.
  Ignatia 6c, every 3–4 hours.
- Stress in tense intellectual types, irritable and touchy, lacking confidence and intolerant of contradiction. Anxiety before any ordeal, such as giving a presentation in front of an audience.
  Lycopodium 6c, every 3–4 hours.

- Stress in active, zealous types, inclined to late nights and rich spicy food, difficulty in sleeping, and desire for stimulants.
  Nux vomica 6c, every 3–4 hours.
- Harassed executives, nervous, agitated and restless, never enough time. Anxiety before meetings; torments from anticipation. Digestive disturbances, seek sweet things, but worse from them.
  Argentum nit 6c, every 3–4 hours.
- Stress in overworked students and professionals, with exhaustion and irritability. Insomnia, sensitive to the slightest noise.
  Kali phos 6x, a tissue salt, every 3–4 hours.

10

The Bach Flower Remedies: Medicine for the Mind and Emotions

The Bach Flower Remedies were developed earlier this century by Dr Edward Bach, MB, BS, MRCS, LRCP, DPH, a physician and homeopath, who spent his life searching for the purest methods of healing. Prepared from non-poisonous wild flowers, the purpose of the Bach Flower Remedies is to achieve a balance between the mind, body and spirit, gently correcting the emotional upsets that give rise to physical symptoms or delay recovery from an illness.

Edward Bach was a physician well ahead of his time. In his short career he moved from orthodox medicine into developing a natural form of medicine to treat emotional and spiritual health, very much in tune with the trends in natural medicine in the 1990s. Bach wrote:

Disease of the body itself is nothing but the result of the disharmony between soul and mind. It is only a symptom of the cause, and it is our fears, our cares, our anxieties and such like that open the path to the invasion of illness. Remove the disharmony, the fear, the terror or the indecision, and we regain harmony between soul and mind, and the body is once more perfect in all its parts.

From an early age, Bach had been aware that people's personality and attitudes have a bearing on their state of health. As a student on hospital wards Bach took an interest in patients as people rather than cases, and early on came to the conclusion that, in illness, personality is more important than symptoms and should be taken into account in medical treatment.

Bach's early medical career was both conventional and successful. In 1912 he qualified at University College Hospital, London, where he became Casualty Medical Officer and later Casualty House Surgeon at the National Temperance Hospital. He also developed a very busy practice close to Harley Street in London.

From 1919 to 1922 Dr Bach worked as a pathologist and bacteriologist at the London Homoeopathic Hospital. There, he learned that Samuel Hahnemann, the founder of homeopathy, had recognised the importance of personality in disease 150 years before. Combining these principles with his knowledge of orthodox medicine, Bach developed seven oral vaccines based on intestinal bacteria which purified the intestinal tract. Bach then made a most important and significant discovery: all the patients suffering from the same emotional difficulties needed the same vaccine, irrespective of the type of disease. From then onwards he prescribed these vaccines according to his patients' temperamental difficulties only. The results were excellent, and these seven vaccines are still used by homeopaths today with great success.

Although the medical profession adopted his vaccines, Bach disliked the fact that they were based on bacteria, and was anxious to replace these with gentler methods, possibly based on plants. He was increasingly dissatisfied with the limitations of orthodox medicine, especially its focus on curing symptoms. Bach closed his laboratory and his lucrative practice and went to Wales to seek further knowledge in nature. Walking through a dew-laden field early one morning, it struck him that each dewdrop, heated by the sun, would be imbued with the healing properties of the plant it lay on. This was the basis of the development of the flower essences.

As he continued his work, his intuition became so sensitive that, by holding a flower or tasting a petal, he could immediately sense what its healing effects would be. He would suffer the states of mind and body for which the flower was needed—a painful and exhausting method of research, but one that gave him a great understanding of his patients. Bach then moved to Cromer, on the Norfolk coast, finding and preparing further flower essences and successfully treating patients with them.

Bach intended the use of the remedies to be straightforward and simple enough for all to understand. The 38 remedies constitute a complete system of healing, each plant having been specifically chosen for its primary function—the ability to treat the mind and restore balance.

Bach placed the Bach Flower Remedies in seven groups, or seven negative mood states which he believed prevented us from being true to ourselves. These cover the entire range of human negative mood states, but each also has a corresponding positive expression.

FEAR: Rock rose, Mimulus, Cherry plum, Aspen, Red chestnut.
UNCERTAINTY: Cerato, Scleranthus, Gentian, Gorse, Hornbeam, Wild oat.
INSUFFICIENT INTEREST IN PRESENT CIRCUMSTANCES: Clematis, Honeysuckle, Wild rose, Olive, White chestnut, Mustard, Chestnut bud.
LONELINESS: Water violet, Impatiens, Heather.
OVER-SENSITIVITY TO INFLUENCES AND IDEAS: Agrimony, Centaury, Walnut, Holly.
DESPONDENCY OR DESPAIR: Larch, Pine, Elm, Sweet chestnut, Star of Bethlehem, Willow, Oak, Crab apple.
OVER-CARE FOR THE WELFARE OF OTHERS: Chicory, Vervain, Vine, Beech, Rock water.

BACH FLOWER REMEDIES

Here are all the remedies and a brief description of the emotional types they are effective in helping.

1 Agrimony

Those who suffer considerable inner torture which they try to hide behind a facade of cheerfulness. They wear a social mask, with repression of sadness.
Positive expression Honest expression of feelings, genuine optimists. Communicate real feelings openly, self-acceptance.

2 Aspen

Have anxiety, apprehension, fear and foreboding of unknown things. Nameless dread.
Positive expression Security and inner protection, become participants in true joy. Inner confidence and fearlessness.

3 Beech

Intolerant of others. Constantly making criticisms. Judgemental. Arrogant. Rigid attitudes.

Positive expression Not affected by others' differences, see good in others despite imperfections. Have desire to be more tolerant, high ideals.

4 Centaury

Weakness of will. Those who let themselves be exploited or imposed upon, and become subservient. Have difficulty in saying "no." Anxious to please.

Positive expression See service as a mutual exchange, are able to express, support and defend own opinions. Serve willingly without denying own needs.

5 Cerato

Those who doubt their own judgment, seek advice from others. Often influenced and misguided.

Positive expression Contact with inner guidance, hold definite opinions, will stick to a decision once arrived at. Quietly self-assured.

6 Cherry plum

Fear of mental collapse. Desperation. Fear of loss of control, of causing harm. Violent impulses.

Positive expression Trust and calm under stress. Quiet courage and inner strength.

7 Chestnut bud

Fail to learn by experience. Continually repeating the same mistakes.

Positive expression Mistakes used as learning experiences, learn from others.

8 Chicory

The over-possessive, demanding respect or attention. Like others to conform to their standards. Control and manipulate loved ones. Make martyrs of themselves. Critical, interfering and nagging.

Positive expression Unconditional love. Able to care for others unselfishly. Sense of their innate capacities. Give without expecting something back.

9 Clematis
Indifferent, inattentive, dreamy, absent-minded and disoriented. Have difficulty in concentrating. Mental escapists from reality. No interest in the real world.
Positive expression Thoughts convert to action, purposeful, realistic. Lively interest in the world. Fulfill their creative potential.

10 Crab apple
The great cleansing remedy.
Feel unclean or ashamed of ailments. Self-disgust, hatred. House-proud, have mental obsession with trivialities.
Positive expression Sense of proportion about problems, become acceptable to themselves again. Control thoughts and deal with difficulties, maintain inner harmony.

11 Elm
Have temporary feelings of inadequacy. Overwhelmed by responsibilities, are over-committed. Feel inadequate to cope. Depressed and exhausted.
Positive expression Self-assured competence, sense of responsibility to self. Problems are seen in perspective.

12 Gentian
Easily discouraged. Pessimistic and have negative outlook. Disappointed and depressed from identifiable causes. Depression from long-term difficult situation, e.g., unemployment, bereavement.
Positive expression Resilient in the face of setbacks, have great conviction. Face life's challenges with courage.

13 Gorse
Despair and hopelessness. Utter despondency—"What's the use?" Feel condemned to pain and suffering.
Positive expression Sense of faith and hope, see light at the end of the tunnel. Will to recover.

14 Heather

People who are obsessed with own troubles and experiences, self-preoccupation. Make mountains out of molehills. Compulsive talkers, poor listeners.

Positive expression Empathy with others, understanding people. Good listeners. Radiate strength and confidence.

15 Holly

For those who are jealous, envious, revengeful and suspicious. For those who hate, are aggressive, bad-tempered.

Positive expression Open-hearted, understanding, tolerant, generous minds, compassionate. Willing to share.

16 Honeysuckle

For those who dwell in the past, with over-attachment to memories. Homesick and nostalgic.

Positive expression Open to present and future. No longer experiencing the past as overpowering, but as a valuable experience.

17 Hornbeam

"Monday morning" feeling, but once started their tasks are usually fulfilled. Procrastinators. Mental weariness, doubt ability to cope.

Positive expression Freshness, strength and enthusiasm. Lively minds, vitality and spontaneity restored.

18 Impatiens

Impatient, irritable, nervous. Want everything done instantly. Energetic but tense. Frustrated by slow workers. Independent.

Positive expression Relaxed, process-oriented, accept differences in pace and style. Cope calmly and diplomatically.

19 Larch

Lack self-confidence. Despondent due to this lack of self-confidence, have expectation of failure so fail to make any attempt. Feel inferior though have ability.

Positive expression Try for personal best, are determined, capable. Aware of own potential with a realistic sense of self-esteem.

20 Mimulus

Fear known things, e.g., illness, pain, accidents, dark, thunder, other people, spiders. Shy, timid.

Positive expression Have no irrational fears, accept life's inherent risk. Anxieties overcome with realism and humor. Quiet courage and confidence.

21 Mustard

Sudden depression: deep gloom that descends for no known cause and lifts just as suddenly. Melancholy.

Positive expression Inner serenity, stability, peace that cannot be shaken.

22 Oak

Brave, strong, determined types whose inner strength wanes; are fatigued. Struggle against adversity despite setbacks. Strong sense of duty.

Positive expression Are stable, strong, patient, full of common sense. Have ability to take it easy sometimes.

23 Olive

Complete exhaustion and utter weariness. Tiredness both mental and physical. All reserves of strength and energy have run out. Lack zest.

Positive expression Restored strength, vitality. Energised.

24 Pine

Self-reproach. Feelings of guilt. Blame selves for mistake of others. Feel undeserving and unworthy. Overconscientious. Never satisfied with their achievements.

Positive expression Self-forgiving, balanced attitude. Renewed energy, vitality and pleasure in living. Responsibility accepted realistically. Accept and respect themselves.

25 Red chestnut

Excessive fear or anxiety for others, especially those held dear. Over-concern for others. Worry about other people's problems.

Positive expression Objective about the welfare of others, calm. Ability to care without anxiety. Radiate thoughts of health and courage.

26 Rock rose

Terror, extreme fear of panic; frozen fear and helplessness; panic after nightmares.

Positive expression Have great courage; are confident, calm. Have strong will and character.

27 Rock water

For those who are hard on themselves, often overworked. Are self-denying; over-concentrated on self. Rigid-minded, their thinking ruled by fixed ideas.

Positive expression Flexible, adaptable. Open to inner truth and willing to change their minds.

28 Scleranthus

Uncertain; indecisive, vacillate between possibilities. Fluctuating moods.

Positive expression Calm, determined, have clear feeling for the right decision. Have poise and balance. Are able to make quick decisions.

29 Star of Bethlehem

After-effects of shocks, mental or physical, as a result of accidents, bad news, deaths, etc.

Positive expression The effects of shock are neutralized. The nervous system is revitalised. Body and soul work together for healing.

30 Sweet chestnut

Agonising mental anguish. Despairing types who have reached the limits of endurance—only oblivion left. Suffer total exhaustion and loneliness.

Positive expression Liberation from despair and depression. Strong characters, resilient, in control of emotions. Have sense of inner support.

31 Vervain

Tense and hyperactive. Over-enthusiastic, put in over-effort, strain. Fanatical and highly strung. Minds race. Desire to convert others. Are incensed by injustices.

Positive expression Calm, tolerant, have ability to relax. Take a broad view of life and events.

32 Vine

Dominating, inflexible, ambitious, tyrannical. Love power. Are aggressive and proud. Have rigid attitudes.

Positive expression Determined without dominating. Have will to co-operate. See good in others and guide without controlling them. Have confidence and certainty.

33 Walnut

Protection remedy from powerful influences, ideas or atmospheres.

Need help in adjusting to any transition or change, i.e., puberty, menopause, divorce, giving up smoking, new home, etc.

Positive expression Have ability to move forward, free of the past; inner knowledge of next step in life.

34 Water violet

Aloof, proud, reserved, sedate types. Have a tendency to withdraw, appearing anti-social and cold. Little emotional involvement. Keep a stiff upper lip.

Positive expression Have independent, comfortable and warm connection with others. Are calm, serene, understanding. Use their talents in the service of others.

35 White chestnut

Have persistent, unwanted thoughts, preoccupation with some worry or episode. Mental arguments go round and round like a broken record. Relive mentally unhappy events or arguments.

Positive expression Have peace of mind, feel calm, constructive. Can let go of worries and unhappy memories and live in the present. Heads are clear.

36 Wild oat

Unable to choose one of many paths, dissatisfied, frustrated. Lack clear direction. Need help in making important decisions.

Positive expression Have knowledge of their intended path in life. Definite character. Clear ideas and ambitions.

37 Wild rose

Resigned, apathetic. Make no effort to change circumstances. Drifters who accept their lot, making little effort for improvement, lack ambition.
Positive expression Passionate, purposeful, lively interest. Their resignation gives way to ambition and sense of purpose. Use initiative to make changes.

38 Willow

Self-pitying, resentful and bitter, with "not fair," and "poor me" attitude. Begrudge others' good fortune. Sulky and irritable, critical. Take without giving.
Positive expression Optimistic, have faith. Responsible for own reality. No longer victims, able to control destiny.

39 Rescue Remedy

A combination of Cherry plum, Clematis, Impatiens, Rock rose and Star of Bethlehem. It is an all-purpose, emergency composite for shock, terror, panic, emotional upsets, stage fright, bereavement, examinations, hospital or dentist visit, etc. Can also be externally applied to burns, bites and sprains. An immediate dose of Rescue Remedy after an emergency can contribute greatly to counteracting its effects and helping the natural process to take its course.

PRESCRIBING BACH REMEDIES

The purpose of the Bach Remedies is to support the fight against illness by relieving depression, anxiety, trauma and other emotional factors that impede healing. They can also be used preventatively at times of high anxiety and stress, and are particularly helpful for those generally unwell and tired, but without any specific medical diagnosis. They take effect through treating the individual, not disease or symptoms of disease. They work specifically on the emotional and spiritual condition of the person concerned. The remedies are intended primarily as a means of self-help, and so self-diagnosis is not difficult.

The descriptions of the states for which the remedies are recommended are not always flattering, and it may be hard to recognize personal traits in them. Bear in mind these are descriptions of extreme states only. All the remedies describe human emotions, common to all, so there is no need to feel ashamed. The fact that they have been recognized is the first step to inner healing. The corresponding positive states will help identify and clarify the correct remedy. As Bach said, "There are seven beautiful stages in the healing of disease, Peace, Hope, Joy, Faith, Certainty, Wisdom, and Love."

The type remedy

In selecting the correct remedy for each person, it is important to choose according to the personality as a whole, so the remedy can be based on a complete picture. The descriptions, both positive and negative, will give important clues in helping determine the particular **type remedy** for each person. This remedy should be used in all prescriptions.

The treatment period of Bach Flower Remedies must be decided on an individual basis, as each person is different and every situation is unique. Generally, however, moods and emotions that have developed suddenly or recently will not take long to correct. Perhaps only a few doses will be required. But for problems that have become deep-rooted and firmly established, perhaps over a period of months or even years, healing will be a much more gradual process and will naturally take longer.

It does help the healing process if it is approached with positive thought, and although this may be difficult in the beginning, the remedies do help the taker to feel more optimistic and thus give hope and lift their spirits. The positive aspect which is strived for—the confidence, courage—is already within us and is re-awakened with Bach Flower Remedies. The remedies do not change the person into someone different, just into themselves again.

Extra remedies in a prescription

When dealing with a particular life problem, emotional states other than those in the type remedy will appear. So at any time the person may have a variety of emotional states operating. These can be prescribed for concurrently, and up to three extra remedies can be included with the type remedy in a particular prescription. When prescribing, it always helps to look for the root cause of the particular problem.

How much to take

Bach Remedies are taken orally, either 2 drops directly on the tongue or 4 drops in a small amount of water which is sipped slowly. The ideal frequency of dose is 4 times daily. In acute cases, such as after an accident or other trauma, the remedies may be taken as often as every 10 minutes.

When to take Bach Remedies

People are most susceptible to the healing influence of Bach Flowers at bedtime and on rising—at these times we are usually most relaxed, and so most receptive. During sleep we also process much of the day's stress, and receive insights from the unconscious. The two remaining doses should be taken as evenly apart across the day as possible, for instance, just before lunch and just before the evening meal. Other times ideal for taking the Bach Remedies are: while having a bath (they may also be put in the bathwater); after meditation and relaxation practices; during therapy; or any other relaxed, secure and open time.

Babies and children

Babies and children can be given Bach Remedies with complete safety and very good results. Children and babies suffer from many emotions and go through times of stress and unhappiness; dealing with these in childhood can help them grow up happily and healthily. The remedies should be chosen in exactly the same way as for adults, whether the child is suffering from a physical illness or is fretful, unhappy or difficult for no obvious reason. The child's personality and current characteristics are the guide to the required remedy or combination of remedies.

Animals

As with children, animals respond well to Bach Remedies. To prescribe, once again, the temperament of the animal concerned needs to be considered, together with its mood and nature generally. Drops of the remedy can be given on food or in drinking water: 4 drops for birds and small animals, 10 drops for larger animals.

Plants

Plants can benefit from the gentle healing properties of the Bach Flowers at watering time, however eccentric it may appear. As plants do not express their feelings or answer questions, their outlook is displayed through their appearance and it is on this expression of need that the remedy is chosen.

Safety

The Flower Remedies are completely safe, have no unwanted side-effects and are non-addictive. They are gentle in action and can be safely taken by people of all ages, from newborn babies to the aged. If a remedy is picked that is inappropriate, there is no threat of harm; rather, the remedy will simply have no effect.

Rescue Remedy

The most famous of all Bach Flower Remedies is the appropriately named Rescue Remedy. As described above, Rescue Remedy is a composite of five Bach remedies. It is a calming panacea that settles nerves, dispels negative thoughts, relieves apprehension and restores balance and confidence. It is ideal for any emergency situation as well as ongoing stressful situations. For example, Rescue Remedy is excellent for shocks, accidents, interviews, exams, speeches, child tantrums, bereavement, dentist or hospital visits, panic situations and mental tension—all common stressors that affect everyone in our society. Rescue Remedy is also ideal for the treatment of hurt animals as often shock and terror is a major cause of their trouble. When transplanting plants, giving Rescue Remedy afterwards reduces the effects of the trauma and helps them to take root again.

HEALING THE MIND

At the end of 1936, Edward Bach died in his sleep, content that his mission was complete. He provided the world with a legacy of remedies to help us if we lose our way, or find ourselves turning back, or if we are uncertain and feel afraid about taking the next step. They help and guide us, but true progress—our real healing—comes from within. Dr Bach's most famous quote probably sums it all up best: "There is no true healing unless there is a change in outlook, peace of mind and inner happiness."

PART THREE

A Materia
Medica of
Common
Remedies

11

Materia Medica of the Tissue Salts

A materia medica is the term used by homeopaths for a collection and description of remedies and how they are used. The remedies listed in the next two chapters have been chosen for several reasons: they are well suited to the sorts of diseases found in the average home, they are safe and easy to use, and they have clear-cut symptoms. Most of the remedies mentioned in the text are included here. The materia medica is divided into two. The first chapter is a materia medica of the tissue salts, which can easily be obtained from most health-food stores. The following chapter lists more mainstream homeopathic remedies.

Homeopathic medicines, including tissue salts, treat the patient as an individual and the body as a whole. Each remedy in this materia medica is summarized, showing the main pattern of symptoms it is used to treat. Often mental symptoms are included, and also the influences that make the symptoms worse or better, otherwise known as the **modalities**. All these combined make up what homeopaths call the **symptom picture** of the remedy.

Remembering this pattern of symptoms for the remedy is the key to prescribing. The remedy that has the symptom picture most closely matching the symptoms of the patient is known in homeopathy as the **similimum**, the most similar remedy, and is the one to prescribe.

In choosing a remedy, there are three main areas for attention:

- the physical symptoms;
- the mental and emotional symptoms;
- the influences that make the symptoms better or worse.

On the other hand, not every symptom covered in the remedy picture needs to be seen in the patient. As a general rule, three good symptoms, characteristic of the remedy and strong in the patient, are enough to indicate the remedy.

Choosing a remedy on just a few physical symptoms alone is the system most prone to error, and often results in the remedy failing in its action. For the best result, the mental and emotional symptoms, such as irritability or tearfulness, should be included as part of the symptom picture, and the choice of remedy reviewed. If, as well, you can include some of the modalities, the influences which make the symptoms better or worse, then you are very close to the similimum, or most similar remedy.

Clearly, to choose a remedy well, the prescriber must be attentive to many small details of the patient's condition which are of no interest to allopathic medicine, with its emphasis on medical tests. In this way homeopathic medicine is perhaps a superior medicine because it is more subtle, treating the person at a deeper level; but it is also more demanding of the prescriber. Small details of the patient's behavior—such as the color of the face, the mode of dress, the way of moving, sitting and lying—can all be symptoms of pure gold to the homeopath.

Since there are many remedies and many symptoms, the ability to know and match symptom pictures is vital, and is probably the greatest challenge of homeopathy. For the beginner, keywords are useful, to draw the strands of a remedy together. These are given at the end of the remedy's description and help as quick summaries of symptom pictures. They are especially useful when a remedy must be chosen quickly.

A more detailed symptom picture of a remedy is also given in the materia medica, and is suited to more experienced prescribers, who are comfortable with remembering symptom pictures.

The ability to remember whole symptom pictures is a highly developed skill. It requires the ability to pay attention to minute detail, but also to recall whole patterns of information, and not everyone has the patience or the will to learn. It is undoubtedly a challenging system of medicine for a prescriber, but if you are interested in the treatment of illness, any effort is well repaid.

Calcarea Fluorica

CALC FLUOR; CALCIUM FLUORIDE; FLUORSPAR

APPEARANCE
The susceptible type is of medium to small build. Teeth are small and irregular, with poor enamel. The skin is hard, especially over the palms of the hands, where cracks and fissures are common. Tongue is cracked.

SYMPTOM PICTURE

■ Methodical and tenacious, with well-organized memory, but easily worried, and preoccupied with money. If a child, is often unstable at school, with poor attention; agitated, undisciplined, a show-off.

■ **Hardening and thickening of tissue**, giving rise to cysts, cystic tumors, ganglions. Hardened **lymph nodes** and **lumps in the breast**, hard like stones. Cataract.

■ Laxness of ligaments and connective tissue. **Visceral and uterine prolapse. Varicose veins. Hemorrhoids**, bleeding, itching and protruding.

■ The bones may be deformed and tender. Scoliosis and sprains are common. Rickets in infants. Callus growths, chaps and fissures of the skin.

■ **Worse Beginning of movement.** Rest. Damp weather.

Better Continued movement. Warmth and hot applications.

Keywords

Lumps

Cracks

Loosens

Sags

Calcarea Phosphorica

CALC PHOS; CALCIUM PHOSPHATE

APPEARANCE

Tall and thin, with tapering hands. Usually dark, with rosy complexion, silky hair and long eyelashes. Skin may be greasy. Teeth are long, narrow and a little yellowish.

SYMPTOM PICTURE

■ **Easily fatigued, especially by mental work;** is hard to finish a long task, even though intelligent. Nervous, agitated and fearful. Memory poor. Sensitive and sentimental; prefers solitude. A good remedy in **convalescence.**

■ **Slow development** in children. Late closure of fontanels. **Growing pains,** at the end of long bones and the dorsal spine. Rickets. Slow-healing fractures.

■ **Glandular enlargements and chronic catarrh.** Tickly cough, with yellow, offensive sputum, worse in cold weather.

■ Colic in infants: vomiting of undigested milk. Severe stomach pains after eating in adolescents. Loss of weight, though eating well. Craving for salt or smoked meat, salt fish. Calc phos improves absorption of other nutrients.

■ **Worse Mental effort.** Humidity. Thinking about illness.

Better Warm, dry weather.

Keywords

Tired

Thin

Glandular

Growing

Calcarea Sulphurica

**CALC SULPH; CALCIUM SULFATE;
PLASTER OF PARIS**

APPEARANCE

Warm-blooded; wants to uncover and be in open air. Tongue has yellow, clay-colored coating, especially at the base.

SYMPTOM PICTURE

■ Absent-minded, irritable, easily angered. **Desires the open air**, is sensitive to draughts, takes cold easily.

■ Torpid **glandular swellings**. Tonsillitis, suppurative stage.

■ Discharges from any mucous membrane; **yellow, thick and lumpy**, often tinged with blood. Eye inflammation of the newborn.

■ **Easy suppuration**; cuts and wounds do not heal readily. Tendency to boils, abscesses and ulcers, anywhere in the body. **Presence of pus, with a vent.** Impetigo.

■ **Worse Wet, cold weather.** Draughts. Warmth of the bed. Exertion.

Better Open air.

Keywords

Thick
Yellow
Lumpy
Suppurating

Ferrum Phosphoricum

FERRUM PHOS; IRON PHOSPHATE

APPEARANCE

The susceptible type is usually tired, pale and anemic. Face alternates between redness and pallor.

SYMPTOM PICTURE

■ A remedy for the **first stage of inflammatory disease**, with fever but minimal exudation. **Mild fever** less than 102°F (39°C), from congestion, heat of the sun or mechanical injuries. Pulse rapid, but weak and soft.

■ **Easy hemorrhages**, particularly nosebleeds. Bright blood from any outlet.

■ **Dry spasmodic cough**, with lancing pains in the chest, worse from cold and lying down. Sputum clear to yellow, often blood-streaked.

■ **Earache**, with heat, congestion and acute pain.

■ **Worse Cold air. Exertion.** Night. 4–6 a.m.

Better Gentle exercise. Warmth. Pressure.

Keywords

Feverish
Anemic
Bleeding
Pale

Kali Muriaticum

KALI MUR; POTASSIUM CHLORIDE

APPEARANCE

A remedy for the second stage of inflammation, with thick white discharges from both mucous and serous membranes. The tongue is coated white or gray.

SYMPTOM PICTURE

■ Acute diseases at the **white exudative stage**. Catarrhal conditions of the **eyes, ears and throat**. Tonsils inflamed, swollen and edematous, with gray pockets. Mumps.

■ Chronic **catarrh of the middle ear**, with blocking of the eustachian tube. Glands swollen. Deafness, crackling in ears on swallowing or blowing the nose.

■ **Thrush and ulcers of the mouth**, with gray—white false membranes, edema and viscous thick saliva. Bitter taste. Indigestion from rich or fatty food.

■ Rheumatic pains with small effusions in the joints, worse by movement and the heat of the bed.

■ **Worse** Warmth. Night. Motion. Open air.

Better Cold drinks.

Keywords

White or gray discharges
Chronic catarrh

Kali Phosphoricum

KALI PHOS; POTASSIUM PHOSPHATE DIBASIC

APPEARANCE

Tired, weak and hypersensitive, with want of nerve power. Tongue clear or coated brownish, like mustard. The eyelids may droop, especially the left.

SYMPTOM PICTURE

■ Excitable, easily angered and obstinate. **Nervous exhaustion**, with dread and depression, especially after protracted illness, emotional upsets or sexual excess. **Fears** the night, falling, people and death.

■ **Cerebral fatigue** and headaches, especially in school children, after **overwork** or mental effort. Loss of memory. Humming in the ears. Vertigo.

■ **Irritability** and hysteria, with alternating moods. Normally **hypersensitive** to stimuli, but may show little response when exhausted. Insomnia. Sleepwalking and nightmares.

■ **Putrid discharges**, from skin or any membrane, with depression and exhaustion. Foul ulcers.

■ **Worse Cold. Excitement.** Worry. Mental exertion.

Better Rest. Open air. Gentle motion. Nourishment.

Keywords

Exhausted
Irritable
Sensitive
Depressed

Kali Sulphuricum

KALI SULPH; POTASSIUM SULFATE

APPEARANCE

Third stage of inflammation, with yellow discharges. Tongue coated; yellow and slimy.

SYMPTOM PICTURE

■ Irritable, obstinate and ill-tempered. **Seeks open air**, even though chilly.

■ **Profuse, yellow or yellow–green discharges**, thin or sticky, from any membrane: may be intermittent and change location.

■ Nasal discharge, yellow, thick and profuse. Loss of smell. Coarse sounds when breathing, with rattling of mucus in the chest, and yellow expectoration.

■ **Scaly skin eruptions**, flaking easily, leaving a moist and sticky surface. **Suppuration**, with yellow or yellow–green discharge. Impetigo.

■ **Worse Heat.** Warm room. Night. Rest. **Better Cold fresh air.** Movement.

Keywords

Thick
Yellow
Suppurating

Magnesium Phosphoricum

MAG PHOS; MAGNESIUM HYDROGEN PHOSPHATE

APPEARANCE

Appears tired and exhausted. May be nervous and thin or emaciated, with rigid muscular fiber. In the acute case will be doubled up, or pacing with pain. Chilly types.

SYMPTOM PICTURE

■ Listless, languid and drowsy; averse to mental effort. Forgetful, unable to think clearly. May stammer and yawn excessively.

■ A great remedy for muscular spasm, often with a sensation of constriction. **Spasmodic pains**, sudden and severe, either cramping or shooting. May change location, be felt anywhere. May be severe enough to cause retching.

■ **Menstrual cramping** that is better after the flow begins.

■ **Abdominal colic**, flatulent and rumbling, no relief from belching, patient must bend double or apply pressure. Renal and hepatic colic. Craves sugar; averse to coffee. May have a thirst for very cold drinks.

■ **Worse Cold**. Right side. Night.

Better Heat. Doubling up. Pressure and massage. Bending forward.

Keywords

Sudden

Spasmodic

Better by heat and pressure

Natrum Muriaticum

NAT MUR; SODIUM CHLORIDE; COMMON SALT

APPEARANCE

The typical patient is pale and thin, particularly around the neck and chest. The forehead may be oily, with eruptions there, around the hairline, and on the sides of the nose. Skin dry and may be cracked, especially the lips and around the nails. Cold sores are common.

SYMPTOM PICTURE

■ **Tired, depressed and pessimistic.** Worries and broods; harbors resentment. Unstable moods, difficult to fix and maintain attention. Easily upset, but **seeks solitude then, and is made worse by consolation.**

■ Takes cold easily, preceded by sneezing. Mucous membranes may be cracked and dry, or discharging. **Discharges watery, copious, often frothy,** and rarely irritating, may be also thick and white.

■ **Eczema or acne** on the forehead, along the edge of the scalp, or in the creases of the joints. **Cold sores** around the lips or anus. Warts on the forehead, the palms of the hands or creases of the fingers. Hangnails.

■ **Craving for salt, or aversion to it.** Excessive **thirst,** or no thirst at all. **Averse to bread, fat,** rich food, meat and coffee.

■ **Worse Heat. Closed rooms. Consolation.** 10–11 a.m. Thunder.

  Better Fresh air. Cold bathing. Fasting.

Keywords

Depressed
Thirsty
Worries
Seeks solitude

Natrum Phosphoricum

NAT PHOS; SODIUM PHOSPHATE

APPEARANCE

May be jaundiced. The tongue is creamy or yellow at the back.

SYMPTOM PICTURE

■ A remedy characterised by **sourness and acidity.** Debility; averse to open air, bathing and company.

■ Catarrh of nose and eyes, with **thick, yellow, purulent discharge.**

■ **Ailments with an excess of acidity. Gout and rheumatism, with cracking of the joints.** Itching of ankles. **Hives.**

■ Flatulence, with **sour risings and sour vomiting.** Jaundice. **Worms;** child picks nose and grinds teeth. Greenish diarrhea. Craves alcohol, eggs, fish, pungent foods. Avoids fat, milk, butter, sour and acid foods.

■ **Worse Mental and physical exertion.** Changes in weather.

Better Cold. Settled weather.

Keywords

Sour

Acid

Tongue creamy at the back

Natrum Sulphuricum

NAT SULPH; SODIUM SULFATE; GLAUBER'S SALTS

APPEARANCE

Often large and fat, particularly over the abdomen, thighs and buttocks, causing the skin to pucker. Skin is jaundiced and dirty-looking. Edema is common. Dirty yellow coating on tongue.

SYMPTOM PICTURE

■ **Weary, sad and depressed**, tired of life, worse at night and in morning on waking. **Great sensitivity to noise**: music may bring irritation or tears. Fears of people, crowds and the future. Results of **head injuries**, may be recent or remote, especially loss of memory and head pain.

■ **Catarrhal inflammation of any mucous membrane**, with discharge either **yellow and watery or green and thick**, but usually irritating, and always worse from humidity. Painful cough, often at the base of the left lung; holds chest with hands. Asthma, worse from damp and 4–5 a.m.

■ **Pain in joints**, especially the lower spine, knees, right hip and ankles, causing restlessness, and often **helped by slow and progressive movement. Warty growths** on skin and mucous membranes. Skin is cracked and fragile, sheds fine yellow crusts; itching while undressing.

■ **Liver painful and congested**; cannot bear pressure or constriction. Appetite poor; averse to meat and bread; intolerant of fruit, vegetables, pastry, cold dishes. Thirst for cold drinks, even though they disagree.

■ **Worse Damp and humidity.** Cold. Near water. 2–5 a.m.

Better Dry weather. Open air. Change of position. Pressure.

Keywords

Depressed
Catarrhal
Edematous
Worse from damp

Silicea

SILICON DIOXIDE

APPEARANCE

Small, thin and neat, though poorly nourished, with clear skin and a good color. The lips crack easily, especially at the corners.

Hands are cold and clammy. Children have a big head and small body.

SYMPTOM PICTURE

■ **Shy, gentle, yielding and polite**; if pressed will become **annoyed, irritable and stubborn.** Conscientious in tasks, but with lack of energy and initiative. **Tired all the time**, with inability to fix attention, even though bright. **Lack of confidence and dread of failure**, with anxiety before any ordeal, but gets through by force of will.

■ **Hypersensitive**, both mentally and physically, especially to noise. **Chilly**, and sensitive to cold and draughts, even when exercising.

■ **Poor resistance to infection**, with frequent colds. Skin is dry and fragile; **suppuration and abscesses are common.** Fingertips are rough; nails are often deformed and brittle, surrounded by septic cracks. **Sweats easily** from the head and feet; foot sweat is profuse, irritating and offensive.

■ **Malabsorption and malnutrition**, yet appetite is usually poor or absent. Excessive thirst is the rule, with desire for cold drink and cold food. Averse to hot foods and meat.

■ **Worse Cold. Damp.** Drafts. New moon.

Better Heat. Dry weather. Rest. Warm clothes.

Keywords

Tired
Sensitive
Sweaty
Suppurating
Stubborn

12

Homeopathic Materia Medica

ere are more than ninety homeopathic remedies. Some of these can be obtained from health-food stores, many from homeopathic pharmacies, and all from homeopathic practitioners. Please consult the Resource Guide at the end of this book.

Aconitum Napellus

ACONITE

APPEARANCE

The susceptible type is robust and vigorous, with an active mind. Often a child.

SYMPTOM PICTURE

■ **Fever, inflammation and pain**, often coming suddenly after exposure to cold or heat, and especially to dry, cold wind. After-effects of shock.

■ **Anxiety, agitation and restlessness**, tossing about, with **greater fear**, often fear of death. Intolerance of pain.

■ Hot, dry, congested skin, without perspiration; but may sweat on covered parts, and on the palms. **Great thirst** for large quantities of cold water.

■ Hoarse, dry, convulsive cough is often present.

■ **Worse   Towards midnight. Extremes of temperature.** Least touch.

Better   Appearance of sweat. Open air.

Keywords

Sudden

Restless

Anxious

Feverish

Dry

Thirsty

Allium Cepa

ONION

APPEARANCE
Not defined.

SYMPTOM PICTURE

■ **Watery discharge** from the nose, **irritating the upper lip**, acrid and profuse. Often begins with sneezing.

■ **Eyes red and burning**, but producing **bland tears.**

■ Irritation spreads downwards to the larynx, and produces a **rasping, tearing cough**, often called singer's cough.

■ Flatulent colic, with rumbling, offensive wind.

■ **Worse Heat.** Closed, warm room. Evening.

Better Open air. Cold room.

Keywords

Nose irritated
Eyes bland
Better open air

Aloe

APPEARANCE

Full-blooded, sedentary people with local congestions. Often women near menopause. May like to eat a lot and drink a lot, especially beer.

SYMPTOM PICTURE

■ **Flatulent diarrhea**, immediately after eating or drinking, or **driving out of bed** in the early morning.

■ Sensation of heat or fullness in the lower abdomen, with constant desire to defecate. **Lack of confidence in the anal sphincter.**

■ Incontinence of feces, on trying to pass wind or urinate. Feces may be solid or gelatinous.

■ Painful **hemorrhoids**, standing out **like a bunch of grapes.**

■ **Worse** Eating or drinking. Early morning. Beer. Oysters.

Better Cold applications. Passing wind or feces.

Keywords

Flatulent
Involuntary
Drives out of bed

Alumina

ALUMINIUM OXIDE

APPEARANCE

Pale, dry and thin, tired and withered, and appearing older than the years would indicate. There may be tremors of the head and limbs. The nose may be sore and cracked at the tip. The eyelids may droop.

SYMPTOM PICTURE

■ **Great fatigue**, mentally and physically. Strong desire to lie down, but worse from doing so. Staggers easily, with **weakness and heaviness of the lower limbs.** Mentally dull in the mornings, brighter in the evenings, although fearful and apprehensive then.

■ **Inactivity of the rectum, with no desire or power:** even soft stool requires great straining.

■ **Intense dryness of skin and mucous membranes.** Skin does not perspire, has a tendency to **crack, itch and burn,** worse from the heat of the bed.

■ Appetite is capricious. May have no appetite, or **may crave indigestible things.** Aversion to potatoes, beer, condiments, onions and meat. Intoxicated by the least amount of alcohol.

■ **Worse Mornings, on waking.** Dry, cold weather. New and full moon.

Better Warmth. Warm, wet weather. Eating. Open air, even though chilly.

Keywords

Dry
Heavy
Exhausted
Constipated

Ammonium Carbonicum

AMMONIUM CARBONATE; A CONSTITUENT OF SMELLING SALTS

APPEARANCE

The susceptible type of fleshy, chilly, indolent and sedentary. Face puffy, skin mottled, pallid or flushed. Looks tired.

SYMPTOM PICTURE

■ **Depressed, prostrated and weak.** Ill-humored and easily upset, especially in **humid or stormy weather.** Faints easily. Sensation of heaviness.

■ Obstruction of the nose at night, must breathe through mouth. Wheezing. **Irritating, incessant, exhausting cough about 3 a.m.,** with sputum difficult to cough up.

■ **Nosebleeds,** when washing face or hands, or after eating. Blood does not clot easily. Palpitations.

■ Gums are swollen, tend to bleed easily. Teeth painful.

■ **Worse** Cold or humid weather. 3 a.m. Menstruation. Water. Ascending stairs.

Better Dry and warm weather. Lying down.

Keywords

Depressed
Heavy
Weak
Bleeding
Cough at 3 a.m.

Ammonium Muriaticum

AMMONIUM CHLORIDE

APPEARANCE

The susceptible type is soft, fleshy and indolent, lacking in reaction. The abdomen is large, the limbs thin.

SYMPTOM PICTURE

■ **Prostration,** with anxiety and irritability. Desire to cry, but cannot.

■ Hot, watery, **corrosive discharge from the nose, irritating the upper lip.** Nose feels blocked. Loss of sense of smell.

■ Constipation, with **excessive wind and hard, fragmenting stool.** Stinging around the anus during and after passage.

■ Sensation of contraction of muscles and tendons, better from exercise. Sciatic pain, worse while sitting.

■ **Worse   Cold.** While sitting.

Better   Open air.

Keywords

Corrosive
Constipated
Contracted

Anacardium Orientale

**SEMECARPUS ANACARDIUM;
MARKING NUT**

APPEARANCE

The susceptible type looks tired, with pale face and dark areas under the eyes. Movements tend to be clumsy. Sedentary types.

SYMPTOM PICTURE

■ **Absent-minded.** Sudden loss of memory, even for recent events. **Lacks self-confidence. Apprehension before any ordeal**, with indecision. Derangements of hearing, smell and taste.

■ **Gastric discomfort, improved by eating**; returns 2 or 3 hours later. Tends to gobble food. Food may taste offensive. Ineffectual urging to stool.

■ Skin pustules or vesicles, with excessive itching and burning. Warts, especially on the palms.

■ **Sensations of a plug or a band**, may be anywhere in the body.

■ **Worse** Empty stomach. Cold and damp. Mental effort.

Better **After eating.** At rest. Evenings.

Keywords

Apprehensive
Forgetful
Better from eating

Antimonium Crudum

ANT CRUD; ANTIMONY TRISULPHIDE

APPEARANCE

Tend to be stout, and may be edematous. There may be cracks at the corners of the mouth and nose. The tongue is often coated white. Patient is chilly.

SYMPTOM PICTURE

■ Great sadness, with frequent tears and absence of desire to live. Impulses to suicide. **Sulky, cross, complaining and disagreeable,** even when kindness is offered. Complaints from disappointed affection.

■ **Burping and regurgitation of undigested food,** not helped by vomiting. **Watery diarrhea** mixed with semi-formed stool. May crave **acid foods and pickles, meat and bread,** which all disagree.

■ Eruptions with vesicles or pustules, especially on the face. Crusts, cracks and ulcers about the mouth and nostrils.

■ **Thickening of the skin:** tendency to corns, warts and calluses, particularly on the soles of the feet. Thick and deformed nails, splitting easily.

■ **Worse** Heat and cold. Overeating. Night. Moonlight.

Better Rest.

Keywords

Sad

Sulky

Thickens

Cracks

Ulcerates

Antimonium Tartaricum

ANT TART; ANTIMONY POTASSIUM TARTRATE

APPEARANCE

No well-defined susceptible type. Generally characterised by prostration, pallor and drowsiness. Sometimes skin has blue tinge around the lips and eyes.

SYMPTOM PICTURE

■ Persistent, irreconcilable ill-humor, worse from consolation. **Prostration, with pale face and cold sweat.** Great **drowsiness**; especially after a bout of vomiting.

■ **Difficult and noisy breathing,** with fine or coarse wheezes. Abundant, ropy, white, sticky, **rattling mucus that is difficult to expectorate.** Suffocative attacks, turning patient blue.

■ **Nausea** may be severe and persistent, relieved by vomiting. Craving for apples and acid drinks, which disagree. Aversion to milk. Salivation is common. Thirst may be absent or intense.

■ Pustular eruptions, leaving a blue–red scar.

■ **Worse** **Damp, cold weather.** Lying down. Evenings. Vexation. Cough worse 3–4 a.m.

Better **Cool, fresh air.** Sitting erect.

Keywords

Drowsiness

Debility

Sweat

Suffocative

Rattling

Apis Mellifica

BEE

APPEARANCE

Face is red, of a rosy or livid hue. Puffy, especially around the eyes. Irregular raised patches and weals in the skin, either red or pale. Patient is restless and fidgety.

SYMPTOM PICTURE

■ Tearful, fearful, fidgety, suspicious and jealous, often after emotional upset or stress. Desires company but not affection. Emotionally unstable and unpredictable, will flit from one idea to another.

■ **Edematous swellings, red or pale**, may be local or general, and may reach both mucous and serous membranes.

■ Burning pricking pains with the edema, **better by cold and aggravated by heat**. Soreness of whole body, sensitive to least touch and pressure. Restlessness, not relieved by motion.

■ **Thirst is absent in edema** and in the hot stage of fevers, but present in the cold stages of fever. Chill is prominent about 3 p.m.

■ **Worse Heat.** Touch or pressure. Right side, spreading to left.

Better Cold. Cool open air.

Keywords

Burns
Stings
Swells
Worse by touch

Argentum Metallicum

SILVER

APPEARANCE

Tall, thin and irritable. Anxious and apprehensive about their health.

SYMPTOM PICTURE

■ **Trembling;** anxious about health. Ailments from anger, fear and fright. Broken-down constitution; **loss of muscular power.** Failing brain power.

■ **Painful hoarseness of singers and speakers. Total loss of voice.** Raw spot over bifurcation of trachea. Cough with easy expectoration of **gray, viscid mucus,** looking like boiled starch. Laughter brings on cough.

■ **Rheumatic inflammations of joints,** especially elbow and knee, after cold, damp weather. Involuntary contraction of fingers and paralysis of forearm.

■ Crushed pain in **testicle,** especially the right. **Ovarian cysts** and tumors, especially the left.

■ **Worse** Using voice. Touch. 3–5 a.m.

Better Open air, even though chilly. Warmth.

Keywords

Weak
Trembling
Hoarse
Depleted

Argentum Nitricum

SILVER NITRATE

APPEARANCE

Withered and old-looking. Emaciation, most marked in lower extremities. Skin may show a blue, gray or brown discoloration.

SYMPTOM PICTURE

■ **Nervous, agitated, hurried and restless.** Lacks self-confidence. Trembles easily. Anxiety before an ordeal. Memory poor.

■ **Vertigo** of heights. **Phobias**, especially of enclosed places and public gatherings.

■ Sensation of **splinters or prickles** in mucous membrane, with **catarrhal discharge. Ulceration** is common.

■ Much **flatulence**, with **violent, difficult belchings. Craving for sweets**, which aggravate. Also craves salt, and may crave ice cream and cold drinks. Often thirsty.

■ **Worse Warmth. Sweets.** Mental work. Stuffy rooms.

Better Cold. Cool, fresh air. Wind.

Keywords

Agitated

Ulcerated

Inflamed

Craves sweets

Arnica Montana

ARNICA

APPEARANCE

Red face and lively expression, or pale and apathetic. Mottled, bruised-like areas may be observed on the body.

SYMPTOM PICTURE

■ Irritable and morose, does not want to be touched. Forgetful and absent-minded, especially after a blow. Great weakness and weariness. A remedy for **shock and concussion.**

■ **Aches, pains and stiffness**, as if bruised and beaten, after too much exercise, surgery, childbirth, or any form of trauma.

■ **Restless**, briefly improved by change in position. Sensation that the bed is hard and full of lumps, will groan, toss and turn.

■ Skin may show **spontaneous bruising**, severe irritation, or eruptions that are mottled, vesicular or pustular. Often symmetrical. Hemorrhage may occur, with dark, venous blood.

■ **Worse   Touch.** Sudden movement or jolt. Damp, cold weather. Heat of the sun.

Better   Rest. Lying with head low.

Keywords

Bruises
Blows
Stiffness
Soreness
Weariness

Arsenicum Album

ARSENIC TRIOXIDE

APPEARANCE

Thin, stylish, neat and well groomed. Meticulous and orderly. Conscious of their elegance, but fragile, lined and drawn. May have a sallow complexion, or be pale. The lower eyelid may be puffy.

SYMPTOM PICTURE

■ **Fussy, fastidious and critical**, easily irritable and peevish. Oversensitive to smell, touch and light. **Fearful** of many things; full of apprehension and dread, especially when alone. Insomnia is common.

■ Weakness and prostration, yet **marked agitation and anxiety between midnight and 3 a.m.**; drives from bed to wander restlessly, even though exhausted.

■ **Burning pains**, like fire, anywhere in the body, but often in the **mucous membranes and skin**, and **improved by heat**. Seeks warmth, and improved by it.

■ Marked thirst for small quantities of liquid, taken frequently. Keeps water by the bedside, but prefers warm or hot drinks.

■ **Worse   Midnight–3 a.m. Cold and damp. 1–2 p.m.**

Better   Heat, except around the head.

Keywords

Burning
Acrid
Restless
Worse around midnight

Arum Tryphyllum

ARISAEMA ATRORUBENS; INDIAN TURNIP

APPEARANCE

Lips dry and cracked, scabs around the nostrils. Patient is restless and irritable, may be prostrated.

SYMPTOM PICTURE

■ **Stinging and burning of the mucous membranes** of the mouth, nose, or throat. May bleed and ulcerate.

■ **Raw, sore throat** of speakers and singers, **worse when swallowing.** Painful hoarseness, with lack of control: voice continually changing, or completely lost.

■ **Clear discharge, irritating the nostrils and upper lip.** Dry lips: patient may chew or scratch until they bleed.

■ Patchy redness or raw hemorrhagic areas may be present on the skin. Lymph nodes may be swollen.

■ **Worse** Heat. Lying down. Cold winds.
   Better Nil.

Keywords

Stings
Burns
Ulcerates
Loses voice

Aurum Metallicum

GOLD

APPEARANCE

Face is ruddy with a puffy, shiny appearance, hair is dark, and so are the eyes. Nose is knobby and red, with prominent veins. The breath may be fetid.

SYMPTOM PICTURE

■ **Irritable and easily angered**, intolerant of contradiction. **Hypersensitive** to smell, taste, hearing, touch, and especially to **pain and cold. Critical of self and others. Suicidal depression**, with lack of self-confidence, particularly for grief or emotional stress. Craves sunshine; finds cloudy days unbearable.

■ **Violent palpitations, with flushing** or congestion in head and chest. Sensation as if the heart missed a beat. Hypertension.

■ **Boring, tearing pains in bones and joints**, unbearable at night. Ulceration of bones and skin. Hardening of glands, especially testicle, with pain and swelling. Uterine prolapse.

■ Increased thirst and appetite, tends to gobble food and crave cold drinks. Desire for coffee. **Craving for alcohol**, and better for it.

■ **Worse Night and on waking.** Noise, Menstruation.

Better Summer. Fresh air and cool applications, even though chilly.

Keywords

Depressed
Sensitive
Critical
Flushed
Craves alcohol

Baptisia Tinctoria

WILD INDIGO

APPEARANCE

The patient is dull and looks drugged, with dusky, mottled face and dark-red mucous surfaces. There may be an anxious, frightened look and facial sweat.

SYMPTOM PICTURE

■ **Great prostration, with fever and mental confusion, may be delirious. Concentration difficult, with drowsiness and languor; falls asleep easily.**

■ **Severe aching pain and muscular stiffness.** Restless; bed feels too hard.

■ All **discharges and secretions**—sweat, breath, urine, stool, etc.—**are fetid.** Abdominal distension. Offensive, debilitating diarrhea.

■ Parched red tongue, swollen and stiff. Constant craving for cold water.

■ **Worse** After sleep. Movement. Pressure. 11 a.m.

Better Nil.

Keywords

Feverish
Fetid
Restless
Thirsty

Baryta Carbonica

BARIUM CARBONATE

APPEARANCE

Both adults and children look prematurely old and withered, with a dried-up, sickly appearance. Children have large abdomens, glandular swellings. Adults tend to obesity.

SYMPTOM PICTURE

■ **Slow to memorize or comprehend.** Vague fears. Easy exhaustion. Childlike behavior in adults. May be physically and intellectually backward. Children slow to walk; timid, easily upset by strangers.

■ **Enlarged glands**, especially the tonsils and prostate. Susceptible to infection, recurrent colds and tonsillitis.

■ Degeneration of the arterial walls. Hypertension from atherosclerosis. **Offensive foot sweats.**

■ **Constant thirst. Avoids cold foods and fruit, especially plums.**

■ **Worse Cold**, from least exposure. Heat of sun. Changes in weather.

Better Warmth. Open air, even though chilly.

Keywords

Weak
Slow
Enlarged
Degenerated
Worse from cold

Belladonna

ATROPA BELLADONNA; DEADLY NIGHTSHADE

APPEARANCE

In acute cases the face is hot and flushed, the pulse full and bounding. Eyes tend to be glassy, pupils dilated. Patient is restless; there may be a furious delirium.

SYMPTOM PICTURE

■ **Sudden, violent onset of symptoms, with restless delirium.** Acuteness of senses: may start at the least noise or touch. There may be hallucination and convulsion.

■ **Intense, throbbing pain and local congestion.** Cramping pains, beginning and ending suddenly.

■ **Fever** with intensely **hot, burning skin.** Hot sweats, especially on the face. Redness of the skin, either in patches or widespread. Measles-like rash, or blister formation.

■ Thirst is not marked, but there may be a craving for lemons and lemon drinks, or a desire to moisten a dry mouth and throat.

■ **Worse Light. Noise.** Jar or sudden movement. Cold air.

Better Warmth. Rest.

Keywords

Hot

Red

Throbbing

Burning

Congested

Sudden

Berberis Vulgaris

BARBERRY

Sickly appearance, with poor color, sunken cheeks and a bluish discoloration around the eyes. The inner part of the lower lip may be livid red, with bluish—red spots at the corners of the mouth. May sit with both hands clasping the head.

SYMPTOM PICTURE

■ Inert, listless, lethargic, with poor memory, and incapable of sustained mental effort. Nervous at dusk.

■ **Prickling, burning, radiating pains,** can be anywhere, but often emanating from the **small of the back,** deeply placed and worse from standing upright or movement. **Cutting pains in the kidney region,** especially the **left,** following the course of the ureter into the bladder and urethra. **Urging to urinate,** with pain and burning. **Renal colic,** with passage of kidney stones or gravel.

■ **Eczema and itching eruptions,** especially when **circular,** burning and smarting, and worse by scratching. Lesions heal from the center outwards. Flat warts.

■ **Acute stitching pain in the liver, sudden and intense. Hepatic colic,** with passage of gallstones. Appetite is variable, with hunger alternating with anorexia, and thirst alternating with thirstlessness.

■ **Worse Movement. Standing upright.** Left side.

Better Rest.

Keywords

Burning
Shooting pain
Worse standing or moving

Borax

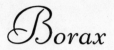

BORAX; SODIUM BORATE

APPEARANCE
Not defined.

SYMPTOM PICTURE
■ Fear of bending forwards, or downward motion. Airsickness. Hypersensitive to sharp and sudden noise.

■ **Ulceration of the mouth and tongue**, may begin as small red vesicles. Worse from touch and salty or acid food. Thrush and mouth ulcers. Baby cannot feed.

■ **Inflammation of eyelids;** margin of lid very sore. Lids stuck together after sleep. Wild hairs; lashes turn inwards and become irritated.

■ Unhealthy skin; every injury suppurates. Vesicles can turn white and coalesce, with a red boundary. **Genital herpes.**

■ **Worse Noise.** Downward motion.

Better Pressure.

Keywords

Hypersensitive
Inflamed
Ulcerated
Herpes

Bryonia

BRYONIA ALBA; WHITE BRYONY

APPEARANCE

The susceptible patient is usually, dark, robust, well-built and well-fed. Face may be puffed and purplish, or jaundiced. Averse to effort, even thought or conversation.

SYMPTOM PICTURE

■ Dry, reliable and tenacious. Methodical and fastidious. Fits of anger and irritability. Fearful, especially about money and the future. Complaints resulting from anger.

■ **Acute, stitching, piercing pains, worse by the least movement,** can be anywhere. Wants to lie still and undisturbed, with pressure on the affected part.

■ **Dryness of all membranes,** both serous and mucous. Dry mouth and white tongue. Profuse sweats, especially about 2–3 a.m.

■ Pain and discomfort in the liver region. Great thirst for large amounts of water, at fairly long intervals.

■ **Worse   Movement. Heat.** Warm weather. The least touch. 3 a.m. and 9 p.m.

   Better   Rest. Pressure. Sweat. Cold.

Keywords

Stiff
Dry
Irritable
Stitching
Worse by motion

Cactus Grandiflorus

CEREUS GRANDIFLORUS; NIGHT BLOOMING CEREUS

APPEARANCE

Face may be red and bloated, pale when prostrate.

SYMPTOM PICTURE

■ Usually sad, taciturn, desiring solitude and made worse by consolation. There may be fear of death and despair of recovery. Tears may be profuse.

■ **Sensation of constriction, as if by wires or a band**, alternately squeezing tighter and tighter, then released; can be anywhere in the body. Pains can be shooting, darting or squeezing.

■ **Constriction of the heart**, with pain down the left arm. **Palpitations**, day and night. **Hemorrhages** from the nose, lungs, stomach, uterus, bladder. Dark blood, coagulating quickly.

■ Hot head with cold extremities. Sudden flushes of heat. Profuse sweats in feverish states.

■ **Worse Heat**. Direct sun. After meals. Lying on left side. Climbing stairs. 11 a.m. 11 p.m.

  Better   Open air.

$\mathcal{K}$*eywords*

Constricting
Palpitating
Bleeding

Calcarea Carbonica

CALC CARB; OYSTER SHELL

APPEARANCE

Often overweight, with soft, pale complexion and lethargic manner. Hands often feel lifeless, lacking grip. Children fair, with large heads. There is often a sour odor to the body.

SYMPTOM PICTURE

■ Well-organized, methodical and economical in effort when well, but **dull, uninterested and easily tired** when ill. Easily discouraged, quickly depressed. Memory poor. Worries easily, with **many fears**. Over-concerned for others.

■ Tendency to catch cold easily. **Chronic catarrh**; enlarged tonsils and adenoids.

■ **Excessively chilly**, with great sensitivity to cold. **Easy sweating of the head**; child soaks the pillow when asleep. Foot sweat, easy and offensive.

■ Digestion weak. **Often constipated.** Averse to meat. Craving for eggs, ice cream and sweets. May crave milk which disagrees. Desire for earth, sand, chalk and uncooked food, in children and pregnant women.

■ **Worse Cold.** Draughts. Wet weather. 2–3 a.m. Exertion.

Better Warm, dry weather. When constipated.

Keywords

Cold
Sluggish
Fair
Fat
Flabby
Faint
Fearful

Calendula

CALENDULA OFFICINALIS; MARIGOLD

APPEARANCE
Not defined.

SYMPTOM PICTURE
■ A remedy with its best action as an **antiseptic wound healer.**
■ The time-honored homeopathic treatment for **cuts and lacerations,** with a particular use in superficial vaginal tearing after childbirth.
■ Also useful as a local application to **diaper rash, sore nipples, burns and scalds, ulcers and infected wounds.**
■ It can be applied as the **mother tincture** in full strength, or diluted I part calendula in 9 parts water without loss of efficacy. It may also be combined with hypericum tincture to form **Hypercal.**
■ **Worse** Not defined.
  Better Not defined.

Keywords

Cuts
Wounds
Rashes
Ulcers
Burns
Scalds

Camphora

LAURUS CAMPHORA; CAMPHOR

APPEARANCE

Pale cold face, with bluish lips and anxious expression. May be prostrate.

SYMPTOM PICTURE

■ A useful remedy for the **first stages of a cold**, with restlessness, chilliness and sneezing.

■ **Sudden collapse**, or sudden sinking of strength, with **icy coldness of the whole body**. Cannot bear to be covered, even though chilly, will throw off blankets.

■ **Sudden shock with collapse. Insect bites, with severe allergic reaction.**

■ Collapse with profuse diarrhea. A good traveller's remedy for **cholera**.

■ **Worse** Cold, yet will not be covered. Motion.

Better Drinking cold water. Warmth.

Keywords

Collapsed

Cold

Will not be covered

Cantharis

CANTHARIDES; SPANISH FLY

APPEARANCE

The acute case may have a red, flaming hot face with staring eyes, or later pallor with a sunken, collapsed appearance. May be restless.

SYMPTOM PICTURE

■ **Intense irritation, both mental and physical.** Confusion, frenzy or delerium, worse by looking at bright objects. Sexual frenzy.

■ **Severe piercing, burning pain in the bladder and urethra**, with frequency and urging to urination. Pains before, during and after urinating. **Urine passes only in drops, tinged with blood.** Pains in the kidney region, radiating along the ureters. Urine retention.

■ Sexual excitation, often accompanied by increased desire.

■ Extreme sensitivity of skin and mucous membrane with **eruption of burning, itching vesicles**, better by cold applications. **Burns, cold sores and sunburn.**

■ **Worse** On urinating. Movement. Touch. Drinking fluids, especially coffee.

Better Warmth. Warm applications. Lying down. Night.

Keywords

Burns
Bleeds
Blisters
Urges

Capsicum

CAPSICUM ANNUUM; CHILLI PEPPER

APPEARANCE

Sluggish and cold, with diminished vital heat, although the face may be red. Looks overweight, bleary-eyed and exhausted. Avoids drafts and open air.

SYMPTOM PICTURE

■ **A remedy** characterised by **inflammation and irritation** of mucous membranes, with an **intense burning sensation** as if a **hot pepper** had been placed on the affected part.

■ It has a particular affinity with the **ear**, and is a very useful remedy for simple **earache in children**, when the whole ear is tender and sore to touch.

■ **Sore throat of smokers**, with pain and dryness extending into the ears. Great thirst, but drinking can cause shivering.

■ **Burning** in all orifices. Bleeding hemorrhoids, sore and stinging.

■ **Worse**   Cold. Drafts. Open air.
Better   Heat. While eating.

Keywords

Burning
Sore
Stinging

Carbo Vegetabilis

CARBO VEG; CHARCOAL

APPEARANCE

The susceptible type is sluggish, pale and puffy, and worn down by debilitating illness. There is a dislike of warmth and a craving for fresh air.

SYMPTOM PICTURE

■ Slow, sluggish and indifferent. **Low vitality**, weakened by illness, loss of body fluids or injury.

■ **Tendency to collapse** from least exertion, with coldness, sweating, pale face, **wants fresh air or to be fanned.** Varicose veins. Puffy hands and feet.

■ **Weak digestion, even the simplest food disagrees. Great flatulence**, better by passing wind up or down, worse by lying down. Craves coffee, acid foods, sweet things and salt. Averse to fatty foods, meat and milk. Intolerant of alcohol.

■ Spasmodic cough, with cold sweat and cold face. Difficulty breathing, with blue–purple tinge to skin, **craves air.**

■ **Worse   Heat.** Being covered. Alcohol.
   Better   Fresh air.

Keywords

Weak
Collapsed
Cold
Flatulent
Craves air

Caulophyllum Thalictroides

BLUE COHOSH

APPEARANCE

Females with patchy pigmentation—moth patches—on the forehead. The upper eyelids may droop.

SYMPTOM PICTURE

■ Chilly, nervous women, especially during **pregnancy, labor and lactation.**

■ **Period pain, irregular and spasmodic**, especially left ovarian region, with bearing down. Thrush, locally and internally.

■ **Labor pains spasmodic, irregular and ineffectual.** Retained placenta. Intense afterpains. Passive bleeding, dark and liquid, after childbirth. Habitual abortion, in the early months, from uterine debility.

■ **Rheumatism of the small joints**, especially the wrist and fingers. Pains are intermittent and erratic, change place every few minutes.

■ **Worse** Pregnancy. Menstruation. Open air. Evening.

Better Nil.

Keywords

Spasmodic
Erratic
Irregular

Causticum

A PREPARATION OF CALCIUM, POTASSIUM AND SULPHUR

APPEARANCE

Usually thin, elderly and tired, with fine, delicate features, grayish pallor. Yellow pigmentation over temples. Eyelids may droop. Trembling may be evident.

SYMPTOM PICTURE

■ Sad, anxious, easily discouraged and depressed, with a peevish and distrustful nature. Intense need for sympathy. **Compassionate: anxious about friends and others.** Ailments from grief, fear, loss of sleep.

■ **Paralysis, especially of face, tongue, throat or limbs. Poor muscle tone of the sphincters:** swallowing difficult, urinary retention or incontinence on sneezing or coughing; constipation with ineffective urging, or complete lack of desire. Hoarseness and loss of voice.

■ **Drawing, tearing pains** in limbs, with **sensation of contraction of tendons**, especially on beginning to move. **Warts**, may be anywhere but especially on face, nose and eyelids, hands, tips of fingers, under nails.

■ Appetite disappears at mealtime; sits down hungry, but smell of food upsets. Craving for smoked and salted meats, beer. Averse to sweets.

■ **Worse Dry cold.** Cold wind and draughts. Twilight. 3–4 a.m. Thinking about problems.

Better Warm and moist. Cold drink improves cough.

Keywords

Raw
Sore
Burning
Contracted
Weak
Trembling

Chamomilla

MATRICARIA RECUTITA; GERMAN CHAMOMILE

APPEARANCE

Susceptible types often have light brown hair and a fair complexion. There may be crack in the center of the lower lip. Babies who are teething, with one cheek red, the other pale.

SYMPTOM PICTURE

■ Children are **irritable, peevish and fretful**, quiet only when carried; want things, but reject them when offered. Adults cannot endure anyone near; are cross, oversensitive, averse to talking. Disorders arising from anger, contradiction or interference.

■ **Oversensitive** to light, noise, smell, and especially to pain; or suffering appears out of proportion to the disorder. Insomnia. Rheumatic pain may drive out of bed at night, to pace restlessly.

■ **Colic** with distension; not relieved by wind. **Diarrhea** of children especially during teething; stool green, watery and offensive.

■ Usually thirsty. Averse to coffee, or intense desire for it.

■ **Worse Anger. Heat.** Coffee. Drafts. a.m. and 9 p.m.

Better Being carried. Warm, moist, humid weather.

Keywords

Sensitive
Irritable
Restless
Hot
Thirsty

China see Cinchona officinalis

Cicuta Virosa

WATER HEMLOCK

APPEARANCE

Face may be pale, with sunken eyes surrounded by a livid ring. When excited the face may be red and covered in sweat. There may be a squint or a staring gaze.

SYMPTOM PICTURE

■ A remedy for **epilepsy** and **tetanus**. Usually of a mild, gentle and placid disposition, may become agitated, suspicious and fearful. Mind may be blank for days.

■ **Violent and intense convulsions**, starting from the head or the face and spreading downwards; after meningitis, trauma or labor. Involuntary urination. Spasms of children, from teething or worms, with distortion of limbs. Before an attack, the child may be excited, singing and dancing.

■ **Yellow pustules**, with honey-colored crusts, especially on the head and face. Eruptions may join together but do not itch.

■ **Abnormal appetite** for charcoal, chalk, raw potatoes and indigestible things. There may be a burning thirst and grinding of the teeth.

■ **Worse   Cold.** Jar or jolt. Trauma.
Better   Warmth. Eating.

Keywords

Spasms
Convulsions
Pustules
Abnormal appetite

Cimifuga Racemosa

BLACK COHOSH; ACTEA RACEMOSA

APPEARANCE
Face pale or bluish, eyes sunken and surrounded by dark rings. Scared, wild expression.

SYMPTOM PICTURE

■ **Restless** in mind and body, can become almost frantic. Cannot sit long in one spot. **Loquacious**; moves rapidly from one subject to another. Fear of imminent disaster, of death, and of going crazy.

■ Complaints initiated by **emotional stress**, disappointed affection or repressed anger. Sudden faintness, with ashen-white face and cold sweat on the palms. Habitual abortion at the third month.

■ **Pains like electric shocks**, darting, shooting and changeable. **Cramping pains in muscles, constantly changing**, with pain and twitching, especially in the nape of the neck, shoulders and achilles tendon.

■ Menstrual pain in proportion to the discharge; **the more blood the greater the suffering**. Bearing-down pains, from one side of the abdomen to the other, causing doubling up, and running along the front of the thighs.

■ **Worse Menstruation. Cold and damp.** Movement after rest.

Better Heat. Open air. Eating.

Keywords

Restless
Changeable
Loquacious
Cramping
Shooting

Cina

ARTEMESIA MARITIMA; WORMSEED

APPEARANCE

Often a child. Pale and sickly, with dark rings around the eyes and pale around the mouth. The pupils may be dilated. There may be twitching facial muscles and eyelids. May yawn frequently.

SYMPTOM PICTURE

■ **Sullen, complaining, disagreeable and irritable.** Adults are touchy, obstinate, no sense of humor. **Child is averse to being touched**, caressed or even looked at; turns away when approached. **May demand things and then throw them away when brought.** Infants want to be carried, or jigged and rocked. **Chilly** and sensitive to draughts.

■ **Bores finger into nose** and picks at nostrils until they bleed. **Sleep is restless**, with jerking and **grinding of teeth.** Tendency to night terrors and urinary incontinence.

■ Convulsions, with urinary incontinence. Teething, chorea (uncontrollable jerkiness), whooping cough and spasmodic affections from intestinal irritation. A remedy for **round or thread worms.**

■ **Intense itching at the anus**, abdominal pains around the navel. Appetite may be **ravenous and insatiable**, with hunger returning soon after a meal. Fussy about food, with many desires. Craves sweet things. Foul breath. Infant may refuse mother's milk.

■ **Worse   Least touch. New moon.** Night. Heat. Full moon.

Better   Movement. Lying on stomach.

Keywords

Worms
Irritable
Disagreeable
Ravenous
Grinds teeth

Cinchona Officinalis

CHINA; CINCHONA BARK

APPEARANCE

Pallor, with sunken eyes, a dull expression and sickly appearance. The face may be puffy, earthy or yellowish.

SYMPTOM PICTURE

■ **Exhaustion**, weakness and irritability from **debilitating discharges or loss of vital fluids.** Averse to company and mental effort; seeks solitude. Anxious and fearful. Intolerant of noise.

■ **Great flatulence**, distending the abdomen, **not helped by belching**, wind or stool. Painless, watery, undigested diarrhea, with marked exhaustion.

■ **Ringing in the ears.** Hemorrhage, from any outlet, especially with buzzing or ringing in the ears, blurred vision, oppression or general weakness.

■ Bitter, salty taste in the mouth. Tongue flabby, coated yellowish–white. Intolerance of acids and fruits, milk and butter, wine and sour things.

■ **Worse   Cold air and drafts.** After eating. Touch. Around midnight.

Better   Heat. Rest. Firm pressure.

Keywords

Exhausted
Drained
Flatulent
Bleeding

Cocculus Indicus

ANAMIRTA COCCULUS; INDIAN COCKLE

APPEARANCE

Fair women and children, of weak and nervous temperament, with weakness, nausea and vertigo. Speech is difficult, and may be slurred. Gait may be unsteady.

SYMPTOM PICTURE

■ **Exhaustion**, with hollow, "all-gone" feeling. Slow in comprehension, seems stupid, or may be very talkative. Bad effects of loss of sleep, emotional trauma, continued worry, overwork, excessive study.

■ **Hypersensitive** to pain, movement, noise and the sight or smell of food. Cannot sleep, even though exhausted. **Vertigo**, with nausea and lassitude.

■ Heaviness, stiffness and lameness in muscles, with numbness and **tendency to tremble**. May stagger on walking.

■ **Nausea and vomiting**, with distension and salivation, especially from motion or pregnancy. Aversion to food: may gag when eating, or even at the thought of it. Thirst for beer and cold drinks. May crave mustard.

■ **Worse Travel and passive motion.** Tobacco smoke. Loss of sleep. Cold air. Pregnancy.

Better Heat. Rest.

Keywords

Exhausted
Sensitive
Dizzy
Nauseous
Trembling

Coffea Cruda

UNROASTED COFFEE BEAN

APPEARANCE

Face tends to be flushed, hot and dry. Excited and talkative, quick movements, or exhausted and unwilling to talk.

SYMPTOM PICTURE

■ Nervous, intelligent and **hyperactive**. Increased mental activity, optimism and euphoria. Easily agitated, may tremble. Rapid changes of mood; can pass quickly from tears to laughter.

■ **Hypersensitive;** vision, hearing, touch and smell are sharper. Oversensitive to pain, tosses about in anguish. Violent palpitations, with nervous excitement.

■ **Sleepless though tired:** ideas crowd into mind.

■ Nervous indigestion, with bloating. Hunger is often excessive.

■ **Worse Sudden emotions.** Stimulants. Cold. Noise.

Better Heat.

Keywords

Agitated
Painful
Sleepless
Sensitive

Colchicum Autumnale

AUTUMN CROCUS

APPEARANCE

Exhausted and trembling, with a waxy pallor. Sits or lies still, to avoid movement.

SYMPTOM PICTURE

■ Great exhaustion; can be too weak to raise head from pillow. **Oversensitive to all impressions:** to light, noise, **smells** and the slightest movement. Excessive irritability; the least thing annoys. May be absent-minded, forgetful and confused.

■ **Swelling of the joints**, with intolerable tearing pains shifting from joint to joint. Acute pains in the **big toe; fears contact or the least movement.** Gout and gouty arthritis.

■ **Very chilly**; feels cold even when close to the fire. Sweating is prominent; may be cold and clammy.

■ Intense **nausea from the sight or smell of food**; may vomit or even faint. Thirst may be excessive, or entirely absent. Abdominal distension with diarrhea and flatulence.

■ **Worse** Movement. Cold. Touch. Nightfall.

Better Heat.

Keywords

Sensitive
Chilly
Nauseous from sight or smell of food

Colocynthis

COLOCYNTH; BITTER CUCUMBER

APPEARANCE

The susceptible type is extremely irritable. In the acute case, the face tends to be dark red, and distorted with pain. Patient may scream, writhe in agony, or double up. May press a hard object into abdomen in search of relief.

SYMPTOM PICTURE

■ **Extreme irritability** and impatience, easily upset by trifles. Disinclined to talk; wants to be left alone. Complaints from grief, anger, and resentment. **Vertigo**, with faintness and weakness; may be too weak to talk.

■ Flatulent distension in the abdomen, with **violent and spasmodic pain**, coming in waves of agony, **improved by hard pressure and bending double.** Vomiting from the pain. **Colic:** digestive, uterine and renal.

■ **Neuralgia**, especially of the larger nerves, tearing and violent, compelling the patient to keep moving.

■ Bitter taste in the mouth, with sore, red tongue. Constant desire to drink fluids. Averse to all foods. Potatoes and cereals are poorly digested.

■ **Worse** Food and drink. Rest. Anger or irritability.

Better Firm pressure. **Doubling up.** Heat. Passing stool or wind.

Keywords

Irritable
Violent
Spasmodic
Better pressure

Conium Maculatum

HEMLOCK

APPEARANCE

Usually elderly and chilly. The face may be flushed, with droopy eyelids. May stagger, tremble or twitch.

SYMPTOM PICTURE

■ Lively disposition, but unable to concentrate or sustain mental effort, moving toward imbecility. **Avoids society, yet dreads to be alone.** Debility after sexual abstinence or excess. Old injuries: never well since.

■ **Slowly ascending paralysis:** movements may be clumsy; walking is difficult, with pain in the legs and loss of strength. Intermittent urination and ineffectual straining at stool.

■ **Intense sexual desire**, unable to be satisfied, or **impotence.** Often **glandular inflammations:** enlarged prostate or ovaries, hardening of testicles, breasts lumpy or painful, particularly the right—often after a blow.

■ Insatiable **craving for salt; great thirst**, and desire for coffee and sour foods. Averse to milk and bread.

■ **Worse** Alcohol. At rest. Touch or jolt. Cold.

Better Warmth. Motion.

Keywords

Trembling
Paralysed
Dull
Strong desire
Craves salt

Cuprum Metallicum

COPPER

APPEARANCE

Face reddish, or red and white in patches. Speech may be impaired. Eyelids may twitch. The limbs may jerk. In acute attacks, the facial skin may be bluish, with blue lips.

SYMPTOM PICTURE

■ Prostration with nervous trembling, after mental strain or loss of sleep. Irritable and emotionally unstable, easily upset. Moods variable; can be depressed or talkative, malicious, fearful.

■ **Spasmodic disorders**, varying from **twitches**, hiccup and **muscular cramps** to violent **convulsion**. Spasms often begin in fingers and toes. Epilepsy, without clear symptoms, or aura begins in knees and ascends.

■ Violent cramps in calves and feet, especially at night, and in the elderly. Dry, spasmodic cough, like whooping cough, with suffocation and palpitation, often worse around midnight. Spasmodic asthma.

■ **Metallic taste.** Desires cold foods. Eats quickly, with tendency to choke. Violent diarrhea, with cramp-like pains.

■ **Worse** Cold air. At night. Touch and pressure. Menstruation.

Better **Cold drinks.**

Keywords

Violent
Spasmodic
Cramping
Better cold drinks

Dioscorea Villosa

WILD YAM

APPEARANCE
Not defined.

SYMPTOM PICTURE

■ A remedy for **pain**, especially in those of feeble digestive powers, with much flatulence.

■ **Severe, acute, colicky pains** that come in waves, twisting and crushing.

■ Griping pains in the abdomen, radiating to back, chest and arms. Sharp pains from liver. **Gallstone colic.** Renal colic.

■ Mouth dry and bitter in morning, no thirst.

■ **Worse Bending double.** Lying down.

   Better Standing upright or leaning backwards. Belching. Motion.

Keywords

Severe
Acute
Colicky
Worse bending
double

Drosera Rotundifolia

SUNDEW

APPEARANCE

In the acute case, there is stiffness, lameness and reluctance to move. Pallor and emaciation may be present.

SYMPTOM PICTURE

■ **Restless and uneasy** when lying down, even though exhausted easily. Sensation of bruised soreness all over, with great sensitivity. Irritated over trifles. Fear of solitude, dreads the night.

■ **Dry, tickling, barking cough**, coming in suffocative bouts; often as soon as the head touches the pillow. Face may become purple; cough often ends in **retching**, sometimes with nosebleed. Holds chest with hands while coughing. Measles, with hoarse cough. Whooping cough.

■ **Muscle pain**, with stiffness and shivering when at rest. Gnawing or stinging pain in the long bones. Always too cold; **chilly** even in bed. Perspires profusely, especially at night.

■ **Hiccups, cramping, gagging and vomiting** characterize the remedy. Averse to acid foods and pork. Food tastes bitter, especially bread. High thirst in fever.

■ **Worse** Lying down. Evening, after midnight. Warmth of the bed. Talking.

Better Pressure of hands. Sitting up. Movement.

Keywords

Restless

Coughs

Tickles

Gags

Worse lying down

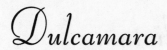

Dulcamara

SOLANUM DULCAMARA; BITTERSWEET

SYMPTOM PICTURE

■ **Restless and irritable**, often with difficulty finding the right word when speaking, and a desire to keep constantly on the move.

■ **Catarrhal discharges** from mucous membranes, especially respiratory, often thick and yellow in the mornings, worse in a cold room or out of doors.

■ **Tearing, shooting or drawing pains**, often coming on during damp cold weather, or after exposure to wet cold, **better by movement** and change of position.

■ Large, soft, smooth, translucent **warts**, usually on the face, the backs of the hands, and the back, where the skin in thin. Sweat is often excessive and offensive.

■ **Worse Damp, cold, rainy weather.** Changes in weather. Rest. Night.

Better Dry, settled weather. Change of position. Warmth.

Keywords

Restless
Rheumatic
Catarrhal
Worse from damp
cold

Eupatorium Perfoliatum

BONESET

In the acute phase, the patient is restless and agitated, and groans loudly with the pain. May be jaundiced.

SYMPTOM PICTURE

■ Adapted to worn-out constitutions, and the diseases of the elderly. Agitation, not helped by movement.

■ Great **soreness and stiffness** of the body, with **intense aching pain in the bones**, as if broken. A good remedy for **influenza**.

■ Coryza (cold virus), with sneezing and aching of the bones of the face. Painful **soreness of the eyeballs.** Cough with sore chest; must support it with the hands.

■ Insatiable thirst before and during chill and fever. Knows chill is coming because he or she cannot drink enough.

■ **Worse Movement**, even though agitated. Cold air. Chill 7–9 a.m.

Better Lying on hands and knees.

Keywords

Stiff
Sore
Aching
Worse from movement

Euphrasia Officinalis

EYEBRIGHT

APPEARANCE

Red eyes and streaming nose in the acute phase.

SYMPTOM PICTURE

■ Acute catarrhal affections of the eyes and nose. Eye disorders, after falls, contusions or mechanical injury. A good remedy for hay fever and sinusitis.

■ Inflammatory **redness of the conjunctiva**, with a sensation of burning. Eyes water constantly. **Irritating tears, profuse and prickling.** Eyelids red, swollen and burning, may be ulcerated.

■ Abundant **discharge from the nose, watery and non-irritating.**

■ Hacking cough, with free expectoration.

■ **Worse   Heat.** Wind. Evenings, in bed.
   Better   In the dark.

Keywords

Red eyes
Irritating tears
Bland nasal discharge

Ferrum Metallicum

IRON

APPEARANCE

The susceptible type is often obese, with a clear waxy skin. Good color over the cheekbones, but mucous membranes are pale. Unstable circulation, pales or blushes easily.

SYMPTOM PICTURE

■ Gentle, pleasant types, but **weak and unstable.** Easily depressed, anxious and weepy, yet irritable when contradicted. **Quickly exhausted**; feel faint on exertion. Intolerant of crowds, pain and noise; seek solitude.

■ Circulatory congestion. **Easy flushing**, frequent nosebleeds. **Very chilly**, feel the cold intensely. Menses pale and watery, with flushes of heat.

■ Muscles **weak, flabby and relaxed**: easy prolapse of the rectum, vagina and bladder. Involuntary dribbles of urine on coughing or sneezing.

■ Craving for sweets, bread and butter; also raw tomatoes and sour foods, even though they disagree. Averse to meat, eggs and dry wine, although sweet wine is well tolerated.

■ **Worse Exertion. Cold.** Night. Heat. Loss of vital fluids.

■ **Better Gentle exercise.** Warmth.

Keywords

Weak
Unstable
Relaxed
Blushes
Bleeds

Gelsemium Sempervirens

YELLOW JASMINE

APPEARANCE

The face is congested, with drooping eyelids giving a drowsy look. Eyes may be glassy, with enlarged pupils. The hands, tongue and eyelids may tremble. Lips tend to be dry and cracked. The tongue is coated yellow–white.

SYMPTOM PICTURE

■ **Prostration. Emotional depression and apathy,** wish to be left alone, but afraid of solitude. Averse to noise and bright light, but afraid of the dark. Jittery and anxious before any ordeal, averse to new undertakings and responsibilities.

■ **First stage of fevers,** of **gradual onset,** with **complete relaxation and lack of coordination** of whole muscular system. **Thirstless,** dull, drowsy and dizzy. **Stiffness, trembling and twitching** in groups of muscles. **Influenza.**

■ Headaches, with disorders of vision, heaviness of the lids and pains in the eyeballs. Pains often located at back of skull, or begin there and spread over the crown of the head to the eyes.

■ Acute catarrhal conditions with watery discharges and much sneezing. Sore throat, puffy, red and congested. Swallowing is painful, with sensation of a lump, or pain shoots from the tonsil to the ear.

■ **Worse** Heat or warmth. Emotional upsets. 10 a.m.

Better Open air. Sweating. Movement.

Keywords

Dizzy
Drowsy
Dull
Trembling
Relaxed
Anxious

Graphites

GRAPHITE

The susceptible type is fat, with a pale, puffy face and heavy features. Lips are pale, and also the hands; skin tends to be harsh and dry. Blushing is common.

Keywords

Fat
Sensitive
Chilly
Constipated
Cracked

SYMPTOM PICTURE

■ **Sensitive, tearful and impressionable**, full of forebodings. Indecisive: dreads effort, both mental and physical. Variable moods: cheerful in mornings, agitated and irritable in evenings. Seeks solitude, but easily consoled. Sleepless, especially in the first part of the night.

■ Circulation poor, with **pallor and chilliness**, sensitive to the least draft of cold air, yet averse to warm rooms and **craves open air**. Enlarged glands and lymph nodes.

■ The **skin is unhealthy**, thick and dry; especially at the fingertips, the orifices, genitals, bends of the limbs, behind ears, on the face and scalp. Lesions **ooze honey-like exudate; may crack, itch and bleed.** Sweats are easy and profuse. Foot sweats and all discharges are offensive.

■ Sluggish digestion, with **stomach pain and flatulence, relieved by eating.** Often has constant urge to eat. **Constipation**, with absence of desire. Craves beer, acid drinks, and cold fluids, which may disagree. Avoids fat, meat, salt, fish, cooked foods. Sweets may cause nausea.

■ **Worse Cold**, except the skin. **Cold drinks.** Damp. Heat of the bed. Night. Skin is worse from warmth, heat of the bed, and washing.

Better Open air, even though chilly. Wrapping up. Rest. Skin is better by cold applications.

Hamamelis
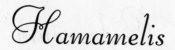

HAMAMELIS VIRGINICA; WITCH HAZEL

APPEARANCE
Not defined.

SYMPTOM PICTURE

■ A remedy with a great affinity for the **veins**. Whereas Arnica is a remedy for injuries where the skin is unbroken, Hamamelis is the remedy for **blows and bruises when the skin has been broken**. It particularly governs wounds when the **blood is dark and oozing**, unlike the fresh bright bleeding of Calendula.

■ It has a particular use in **dilated, sensitive and painful veins**, with a sensation of **bruised soreness** and **fullness** as if they may burst. Hence it has great use in **varicose veins in the legs**, particularly during pregnancy, after childbirth, or after standing for long periods.

■ **Hemorrhoids**, sore and bruised, after pregnancy or childbirth.

■ **Nosebleed**, especially in the morning, with thin, dark blood.

■ **Worse** Cold. Drafts. Open air.

Better Heat. While eating.

Keywords

Bruised and bleeding
Sore and full
Thin, dark blood

Hepar Sulphuris Calcareum

HEPAR SULPH; HAHNEMANN'S CALCIUM SULPHIDE

APPEARANCE

Fair, scrawny and torpid, sensitive to cold. Face often has a yellow tinge. The lower lip may be cracked. Skin has an unhealthy look.

SYMPTOM PICTURE

■ **Oversensitive** to all impressions, especially pain and cold. Quarrelsome and **easily angered**, irritable from the slightest cause, intolerant of contradiction. Memory is poor. Speaks quickly, dislikes fuss, and prefers solitude.

■ **Easy infections** of all respiratory membranes. Laryngitis, with loose, raucous, noisy cough, worse from cold air. **Croup.** Chronic enlargement of the tonsils, with easy infection. Painful sensation in the throat, as if a **splinter or needle** is stuck there. Sneezing and blocked nose in open air.

■ Skin easily cracks and chaps, and shows eruptions, cold sores, boils and ulcers. Even **small injuries suppurate**, become septic and offensive, **hypersensitive to pain, touch and cold air**; contact with clothing is painful, and the slightest draft is not tolerated. Sweat tends to be easy and profuse, especially at night; often sour and offensive, and does not relieve.

■ Craving for vinegar, pickles, alcohol, condiments. Averse to fat foods. Faint feeling with hunger occurs mid-morning. There may be excessive thirst.

■ **Worse** Cold. Cold wind and drafts. Touch.

Better Warmth. Damp weather.

Keywords

Sensitive
Suppurates
Splinters
Cracks

Hypericum Perforatum

ST JOHN'S WORT

APPEARANCE

The expression may be one of suffering due to severe pain at the time of injury, or persisting after it.

SYMPTOM PICTURE

■ **Severe depression** following injury, involving either peripheral or nervous tissue. Consequences of fright and shock. Impairment of memory, and tendency to make mistakes in writing. Drowsiness may be marked.

■ Trauma to nerve endings, from crushing, laceration, puncture or bruising, and especially after dental extraction, surgery or amputation. Excessive soreness and tenderness of injured parts, with **shooting, tingling or burning, lightning-like pains** that come and go and may be accompanied by numbness.

■ Spinal disorders with extreme sensitivity of vertebrae. Twitching of the muscles. Following blows to the coccyx. Brain and spinal concussion.

■ There may be a craving for wine. Desire for warm drinks is recorded, also intense thirst in association with trembling.

■ **Worse Cold and damp. Touch.** Jar. Motion.

Better Rest. Bending head backwards.

Keywords

Crushed
Punctured
Nervous
Shooting

Ignatia Armara

STRYCHNOS IGNATII; ST IGNATIUS BEAN

APPEARANCE

Often female. Face changes color frequently, from pale to flushed at the least emotion. Sighs, twitches and yawns.

SYMPTOM PICTURE

■ **Sensitive**, refined dispositions, quick to perceive, rapid in execution. May be physically exhausted from long-endured grief, anxiety or emotional shock. Grieves silently and seeks solitude.

■ **Unstable** mental and emotional states, rapidly **alternating, contradictory** and extreme. High emotional tension. Sighs or yawns often, or shows **spasmodic affections** such as spasms, cramps, twitches, tics or hiccups.

■ Oversensitive: emotionally, mentally and physically. Cannot endure strong smells, especially coffee and tobacco. Hypersensitive to pain.

■ **Contradictory in appetite:** averse to ordinary diet, warm food and meat, but may crave indigestible or exotic foods. Empty feeling in stomach, not relieved by taking food. Sore throat not worse by swallowing solids.

■ **Worse Grief, worry and guilt.** Stimulants. Strong odors.

Better When the mind is occupied. Warmth.

Keywords

Sensitive
Sad
Spasmodic
Changeable
Contradictory

Iodum

IODINE

APPEARANCE

Often dark-haired and swarthy, usually thin. The face tends to be flushed, the expression anxious and excited. The speech is careful, with attention to detail. Lymph nodes and thyroid may be enlarged.

SYMPTOM PICTURE

■ **Extreme weakness**, with palpitation, **hot flushes** and trembling. Anxious, apprehensive and impulsive. Zealous, intense types, **never still**, must always be doing something. Uneasy sleep.

■ **Glands enlarged or atrophied**, especially thyroid, testes and breasts. **Intolerant of heat**, with **sensation of always being too hot**; constantly seek cooler surroundings. Sudden, profuse hot sweats; acrid foot sweats.

■ Catarrhal affections of all mucous membranes, expecially mouth and throat. Mouth ulcers. Laryngitis, with wheezing cough, dry, suffocating and croup-like.

■ **Ravenous hunger** every few hours, or loss of appetite, but remain **thin and debilitated even though eating well**. Abdominal distension with loud belching and gurgling. Excessive salivation, with soapy or salty taste. Crave meat and alcohol. Intolerance of milk.

■ **Worse   Heat. Humidity.** Exertion. 3–4 a.m.

Better   Eating. Open air. Fully occupied.

Keywords

Hot
Weak
Hungry
Anxious
Restless

Ipecacuanha

IPECAC; CEPHAELIS IPECACUANHA

APPEARANCE

In the acute case the face is pale, drawn and nauseated, with dark rings around the eyes. The tongue is clean, or only slightly coated. Shuddering may be prominent.

SYMPTOM PICTURE

■ Extreme impatience, with morose irritability and discontent. Children wail and scream continuously; adults are sulky and ill-humored. There is a **great sensitivity to noise. Excessive chilliness**; the slightest cold is unbearable. May be called for in complaints arising from vexation.

■ **Sudden, violent and persistent nausea, not improved by vomiting, accompanies many complaints.** Salivation is excessive. **Hemorrhage may be present. The vomit is tenacious, white, abundant, may be bloody, accompanied by rapid exhaustion, yawning and shuddering.**

■ **Wheezing, spasmodic, suffocative cough,** accompanied by nausea and sometimes the vomiting of phlegm. Accumulation of rattling mucus in the bronchi, yet nothing can be brought up. **Nosebleeds** are common.

■ Lack of appetite and thirst, and **aversion to all food**, especially veal or pork. Dysentery-like stools, may be viscous, watery and bloody, with nausea and ineffectual urging.

■ **Worse   Cold.** Heat. Food.

Better   Firm pressure. At rest, with eyes closed. Warmth.

Keywords

**Nausea not relieved by vomiting
Excess salivation**

Kali Bichromicum

KALI BICH; POTASSIUM BICHROMATE

APPEARANCE

Fat, chilly and blond, predisposed to catarrh. The complexion may be sallow or florid. Chronic cases may be emaciated. Tongue is yellow and coated at the base, or glazed, red and cracked.

SYMPTOM PICTURE

■ Drowsiness, with prostration. Ill-tempered, low-spirited and listless. Averse to effort and to meeting strangers. Memory is poor, with a tendency for thoughts to vanish. **Chilly**, and likes to be well wrapped up.

■ **Tenacious, yellow or yellow–green discharges** from any mucous membrane, **may be ropy or jellylike.** Nasal discharge forms crusts. Chronic sinusitis. **Ulceration of mouth, inside nose, throat, stomach and skin,** with sharp, burning pain.

■ **Rheumatic pains, shifting from joint to joint.** Sciatic pains that come and go suddenly, and shoot down the limb, made better by movement. Pains in the soles of the feet, and especially the heels.

■ Pain, wind and **burning in the gastric region** from inflammation or ulceration. Nausea and vomiting after meals, sudden, yellow and bitter. Aversion to water, potatoes and coffee. Desire for beer and acid drinks even though poorly tolerated.

■ **Worse Cold.** Cold winds. Undressing. 2–4 a.m.

Better Warmth. Movement. Firm pressure.

Keywords

Thick
Yellow and tenacious
Plugs
Ulcerates

Kali Carbonicum

POTASSIUM CARBONATE

APPEARANCE

Face pale or jaundiced: soft, swollen and flabby looking, with red nose. Bag-like swelling between eyebrows and lids, with edema of the internal angle. May be obese.

SYMPTOM PICTURE

■ **Anxious, nervous, fearful and hypersensitive**, starting at the least noise and the least touch. Excessively ticklish. **Easily discouraged**, may weep when telling symptoms, and tends to exaggerate them. Averse to solitude, wants company but not sympathy.

■ **Great debility with profuse sweats on slightest exertion**, often with constant, weary backache. **Chilly**, with feeble circulation: shivers often; takes cold easily. Asthmatic attacks **2–4 a.m.**, better by bending forwards; coughing up of small gray lumps.

■ **Stabbing pains**, cutting and burning, **coming at any time** and can be anywhere, worse by pressure, and independent of movement; **may cry out suddenly.**

■ **Impaired digestion, with excessive flatulence and colic**, especially after eating, even when meals are light. Abdomen sensitive to touch. Intense desire for sweet or sour foods. Averse to cabbage, hot food and milk.

■ **Worse Cold. 2–4 a.m. Right side.** Touch and pressure. Outdoors.

Better Warm room. Warm, moist weather. Daytime.

Keywords

Anxious
Nervous
Fearful
Sensitive
Sudden pains

Lachesis Mutus

VENOM FROM THE BUSHMASTER SNAKE

APPEARANCE

The susceptible type has a bluish, congested appearance to the nose, cheeks and ears; a network of small veins may be visible there. Hair may be reddish brown. Expression is anxious, suspicious, even furtive.

SYMPTOM PICTURE

■ **Periods of despondency**, with depression and anxiety, **alternating with excitement. Very talkative**, wanders easily from the point. Can be **suspicious, jealous** and **obsessive**, proud and vindictive.

■ Great **sensitivity** of all senses to stimuli, but particularly **touch and noise. Fears constriction**, even of clothing, especially about the throat and waist. Always **better from the appearance of discharges.**

■ Unstable circulation. **Hot flushes**, particularly around menopause. Spontaneous bruising after the smallest trauma.

■ **Tongue trembles**, is difficult to protrude. Thirst may be insatiable. Desire for alcohol, milk and oysters. Averse to bread and hot drinks.

■ **Worse Tight clothing. Before discharges. During and after sleep.** Heat. Left side. Night.

Better Appearance of discharges. Mild temperature. Open air.

Keywords

Fears constriction
Sleeps into aggravation
Better from discharges

Ledum Palustre

LABRADOR TEA

APPEARANCE

Robust, florid, gouty individuals. Congested face, with red spots on the cheeks and forehead. Pupils may be dilated. May be alcoholic.

SYMPTOM PICTURE

■ Cross and peevish, discontented with everybody. Everything is disagreeable. **Chilly, but wants cold for relief.** Restless and sweaty at night, finds heat of the bed intolerable, throws off the covers.

■ **Injuries** due to **sharp instruments**, or **puncture wounds** that do not bleed, such as **insect bites.** The skin is swollen, pale and mottled, and the pain is local.

■ **Painful swellings of the joints, hot but pale**, and **better by cold applications.** May start in the feet and spread upwards. Pain is tearing, pulling or stabbing, may shift rapidly. Gouty swelling of the big toe.

■ **Bruises**, especially when burning black. **Black eyes.** Hemorrhages; may be bright red, but often dark.

■ **Worse Movement. Warmth.** Pressure. Night.

Better Cold. Cold applications. Rest.

Keywords

Hot
Pale and swollen
Better by cold
Black and bruised

Lilium Tigrinum

TIGER LILY

APPEARANCE

Usually nervous, fair and fat, with poor color and a wild look in the eye. Listless and inert, yet cannot keep still. Tongue may be coated yellow—white in patches.

SYMPTOM PICTURE

■ **Depressed, hurried and worried**, with easy crying and desperation. **Exacting, irritable and hypercritical:** almost impossible to please. Many fears, including solitude, but made worse by consolation.

■ **Intense pressing down in vagina, bladder and rectum**, as if the pelvic organs were heavy and could fall out, worse before menses; must sit down, wants support. Pressure in the rectum: **constant desire for stool and urination.** Menstrual flow only when moving about, and in the daytime. **Increased libido, especially before menses.**

■ Sensation of **constriction of the heart, as if grasped by a hand**, with palpitation and radiation down the right arm, helped by lying on the left side.

■ May remain hungry, in spite of having a good meal. Thirst may be excessive. May crave or be averse to meat; also may be averse to bread, coffee and smoking. Cannot stand a belt about the waist.

■ **Worse Heat. Standing.** Closed rooms. Consolation.

  Better Cool. Open air.

Keywords

Depressed
Hurried
Worried
Bearing down
Worse heat

Lycopodium

SPORES OF THE CLUB MOSS; LYCOPODIUM CLAVATUM

APPEARANCE

Often professional types. Face is intelligent but sallow and lined, with a worried expression; there may be a marked vertical frown above the root of the nose. Dark hair graying early; looks older than really is. Body may be thin and poorly developed; may stoop.

SYMPTOM PICTURE

■ **Intellectually keen but physically weak.** Anxious, irritable and difficult. Authoritarian and reserved, **dislikes contradiction. Lacks self-confidence:** averse to starting new undertakings, **apprehensive before any ordeal. Many fears:** of crowds, dark, death, strangers. Likes solitude but dislikes being entirely alone. **Sensitive to cold, smells and noise.**

■ Disorders of mucous membranes everywhere, especially throat, lung and genito-urinary. Gets colds and sore throats easily. **Right-sided symptoms,** or symptoms go from right to left.

■ Appetite moderate or ravenous, but **may be satiated after only a few mouthfuls. Flatulent dyspepsia and bloating** after meals—must loosen waistband—and are not helped by belching or passing wind. Constipation without desire, from disorganization of the sphincters.

■ **Craves sweet foods and hot drinks. Averse to cold food, onions,** meat, coffee, cabbage, beans and starchy foods. Oysters disagree.

■ **Worse 4–8 p.m. Cold.** On waking in morning. Right side. Contradiction.

Better Fresh air. Movement. Hot food and drink.

Keywords

Intellectual

Fearful

Flatulent

Bloated

Craves sweets

Mercurius Solubilis

HAHNEMANN'S SOLUBLE MERCURY

APPEARANCE

Flabby with sickly complexion. The tongue is moist and flabby, coated yellow or white, and shows the imprint of the teeth. Offensive breath may be obvious.

SYMPTOM PICTURE

■ **Great debility**, of mind and body. **Easily exhausted**, yet is restless, agitated and anguished, especially at night. Memory and will power are impaired. Chilly and sensitive to changes of temperature, but worse by both heat and cold.

■ **Discharges** from any mucous membrane, **yellow–green, irritating and offensive**, especially eye, nose, throat, lung and genitals, leaving skin raw and irritated. Membranes may ulcerate, especially the mouth and throat.

■ **Offensive sweat, greasy or abundant**, especially at night, without relief.

■ **Foulness of the mouth**, with offensive breath. **Excessive salivation, with marked thirst**, may wet the pillow during sleep. Craves stimulants; averse to meat, fat and butter.

■ **Worse Night. Heat. Heat of the bed. Cold.** Wet and damp. Drafts.

Better Rest. High altitude.

Keywords

Stinks
Sweats
Salivates
Ulcerates
Worse at night

Mezereum
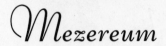

DAPHNE MEZEREUM; SPURGE OLIVE

SYMPTOM PICTURE

■ Irritable over trifles, averse to everything. Takes no pleasure in anything. Forgetful while speaking, may lose the thread. Drowsy during the day, sleep at night is restless and broken. Chilly, with cold hands and feet, even in a warm room.

■ **Burning pains in the bones of the nose and face**; mucous membranes may ulcerate. Sinuses painful. Sneezing, with yellow discharge that may be streaked with blood. Sudden edema. There may be loss of smell, deafness and tinnitus.

■ **Violent itching of skin**, even without lesions, changing location and made worse from scratching and the heat of the bed. **Intolerably itchy, burning vesicles**, cloudy or purulent, with **severe neuralgia** in affected area. Lesions mature into ulcers with yellow pus, covered by a thick white crust. Impetigo, eczema, herpes and shingles.

■ Intense burning in mouth, throat and stomach, relieved temporarily by food or milk. May crave fat, especially ham. Flatulent colic. Digestive mucosa may ulcerate.

■ **Worse** Cold. Damp. Humidity. Touch. Night. Heat of bed.

Better Open air.

Keywords

Violent
Burning
Itching
Painful
Erupting

Natrum Carbonicum

NAT CARB; SODIUM CARBONATE DECAHYDRATE

APPEARANCE

Anemic, emaciated type, with pale face and blue-ringed eyes.

SYMPTOM PICTURE

■ **Great debility**; cannot think or exert easily. Depressed, irritable, melancholic and apprehensive, seeks solitude. **Hypersensitive** to noise and music. **Body and limbs sensitive to cold; head sensitive to warmth** and the heat of the sun, will bring **headaches**.

■ **Visceral prolapse. Menstrual bearing down**, as if everything would come out. **Joints weak and delicate**; turn and sprain easily.

■ Chronic catarrhal conditions of all mucous membranes, with **copious yellow–green mucus**, thick and often offensive. Worse in the day and from drafts, better from sweating. Cough sore, loose and chronic; supports chest with hands.

■ **Gastric discomfort, with frequent belching, great acidity** and large appetite, **worse 10 or 11 a.m.** Loves sweets and nibbling. Diarrhea, with urgent desire, yellow like pulp of an orange. Averse to vegetable diet and starchy foods. Averse to milk; causes diarrhea.

■ **Worse Warm weather. Heat. Cold.** Music. Mental work. Storms.

Better Eating. Movement.

Keywords

Weak and debilitated
Body fears cold
Head fears heat

Nitricum Acidum

NITRIC ACID

APPEARANCE

The typical patient usually has dark hair and eyes, and a pale or sallow complexion. The face is often deeply lined; eyes may be dull, with large pupils. Likely to be thin or emaciated. Tongue may be mapped, like ringworm on sides.

SYMPTOM PICTURE

■ **Great debility with lack of stamina**, but can be very obstinate. **Depressed and anxious**, especially in the evening. **Oversensitive** to noise, pain, touch or jar. Easily irritated, can be vindictive. **Indifferent**, and intolerant of sympathy.

■ **Pricking, sticking pains** as if from splinters, can be anywhere, but mostly in **bone, throat, nose and anus**, worse from contact, movement, or swallowing. Profuse and offensive **discharges from skin and mucous membranes**, thin and stinging, perhaps dirty yellow–green.

■ **Cracks, fissures, warts and ulcerations on the orifices**: skin may be yellow there. **Sweats easily** from hands and feet even though chilly, and especially after midnight.

■ Craving for fats and fatty foods, which will often aggravate. Often a craving for salt, chalk, lime and earth. Bread may disagree.

■ **Worse Cold. Wet.** Wind. Thunder. **Fats**, even though often craved.

Better Smooth motion, such as riding in a car.

Keywords

Depressed
Debilitated
Ulcerated
Cracks
Prickles

Nux Vomica

STRYCHNOS NUX-VOMICA; POISON NUT

APPEARANCE

Generally lean and active, hearty and full of life. Sallow complexion, lined face and dark shadows under the eyes. Often business types and sedentary brain workers, overloaded with work and responsibility. Usually male.

SYMPTOM PICTURE

■ **Irritable, nervous and chilly. Oversensitive** to noise, light, smells, and cannot bear contradiction. Fastidious and methodical. Active and sociable in the evening, seeks strong enjoyments and late hours. In morning **wakes tired and irritable**; seeks stimulants to start the day. Overwork, with depression and suicidal tendencies. A remedy for hangovers.

■ **Insomnia around 3–4 a.m.** May sleep again just before dawn; wakes tired and unrefreshed.

■ **Habitual constipation**, frequent but inefectual desire for stool, passes but a little at each attempt. Hemorrhoids are common, helped by cold applications.

■ Gastric **discomfort 1–2 hours after a meal**, must loosen clothes. Sleepy after meals, cannot work then; a short nap improves. Craves **alcohol, rich or spicy foods and coffee.** Averse to meat, milk, bread and cold food.

■ **Worse** In morning on waking. 3–4 a.m. Mental effort. Cold.

  Better Warmth. Rest. Damp weather.

Keywords

Irritable
Sensitive
Craves stimulants
Worse mornings

Petroleum

COAL OIL

Thin, fair, cold sensitive, and nervous, with a dry and dirty skin.

SYMPTOM PICTURE

■ Irritable and quarrelsome; trifles offend. Vivid imagination.

■ **Motion sickness**, with nausea and vertigo, better by closing the eyes. Nausea in the morning, with accumulation of water in the mouth.

■ **Skin is dry, thick, rough, cracked**, sore and bleeding; easily infected, and **worse in winter** and after washing. Fingertips chap and crack easily in winter. Sweats are foul. Heat and burning of the soles and palms.

■ Gnawing sensation in stomach, better by constant eating. Intense hunger and thirst, but does not gain weight. Craves beer. Cannot eat cabbage or sauerkraut.

■ **Worse   Winter. Cold.** Motion. Storms. **Better   Summer. Heat.**

Keywords

Nauseous
Skin dry and cracked
Worse motion and
winter

Phosphoricum Acidum

PHOSPHORIC ACID

Haggard and worn out. May be young, tall and thin, growing fast. The face is pale and pinched, with blue rings around the eyes. The pupils may be unequal and the eyes have a glassy look. The hair may be prematurely gray and sparse.

SYMPTOM PICTURE

■ **Exhaustion with apathy**, after loss of vital fluids, severe emotional upsets, stress or overwork. **Listless, chilly and indifferent**, although oversensitive to music and odors. Premature hair loss with mental depression and muscular weakness.

■ **Weakness of memory**; cannot think, connect ideas or find the right words. Tired during the day, sleepless at night. Headaches with pressure on the crown of the head, often after intellectual work in students, eyestrain or sexual intercourse.

■ **Abundant urine**, may be clear or milky, especially at night.

■ Acute or chronic **diarrhea—abundant, watery, painless and odorless**—which is not exhausting, and may improve other symptoms. Great thirst for cold milk and beer. Averse to bread and coffee.

■ **Worse** Physical or mental effort. Sexual excess. Least draft. Cold.

Better Warmth. Sleep. Walking.

Keywords

Exhausted
Apathetic
Excessive urine and diarrhea

Phosphorus

PHOSPHORUS, THE ELEMENT

APPEARANCE

Tall and slender, with a narrow chest. May have either dark hair, brown eyes and long eyelashes, or fair skin, freckles and fine hair either blond or red. Often blue rings and much puffiness around the eyes, and a general sickly, waxy appearance. Restless, with fidgety hands.

SYMPTOM PICTURE

■ **Artistic, imaginative, sensitive and creative. Anxious, especially around sunset**, and full of fears. **Easily exhausted** by stimuli: alternates between excitement and depression. **Craves company, attention and affection**; may be lively and talkative, or silent and indifferent.

■ **Chilly**, but with **sensations of burning in spots**, particularly between the shoulders, but can be anywhere. Heat may run up the spine into the head. Profuse sweats on exertion, or in bed.

■ **Easy bleeding**, frequent and abundant from any mucous membrane. **Ulceration** is common. Hard, dry, tight cough, with bloody sputum. Easy flushing.

■ **Craves cold food and drink, salt**, sour and spicy food. Averse to sweet foods, milk, tea, meat, salt fish and oysters. Hunger around 3 a.m., may drive from bed to eat. Great thirst for cold water.

■ **Worse Cold, except head and stomach. Storms. Twilight. Lying on the left side.** Damp and humidity.

Better Warmth. Sleep, even a short nap. On eating. Massage.

Keywords

Burns
Bleeds
Exhausted
Ulcerates
Fidgets

Phytolacca Decandra

POKEROOT

Pale face, becoming flushed after eating. Skin is dry, and may have a leaden hue.

SYMPTOM PICTURE

■ Gloomy, with fear of death. Shamelessness and lack of delicacy may be apparent.

■ **Dark red, painful swelling of the throat,** and sensation of foreign body that cannot be swallowed. Pain from the root of the tongue to the ears, worse from heat and swallowing. Uvula (flap of skin at back of throat) may be swollen and transparent.

■ **Congestions of the breasts, with stony hard, painful nodules.** Mastitis. Nipples may inflame and crack; pain radiates to whole of the body.

■ Sensations of **stiffness, soreness and bruising all over body; desires to move but aggravated by it.** Rheumatic and neuralgic **pains in bones and fibrous tissue, burning and shooting**, may shift rapidly, or come and go suddenly. **The neck** is particularly liable to be affected.

■ **Worse** Cold, especially **damp cold. Night. Movement**, despite restlessness.

Better Dry weather. Warmth. Rest.

Keywords

Stiff
Sore
Bruised
Restless
Worse motion

Psorinum

APPEARANCE

The susceptible type is thin to the point of emaciation, with a pale, ill appearance, a sharp, long nose, a long upper lip and large ears. Usually well wrapped up. Skin is dirty-looking, dry or greasy, with a mousy odor. Hair is unkempt, despite combing.

Keywords

Depressed

Thin

Chilly

Skin worse heat and washing

SYMPTOM PICTURE

■ **Depressed metabolism, with weakness** and lowered vitality. **Depressed mentality**; pessimistic and introverted, cannot stand noise, seeks solitude. **Anxious, with many fears**: of the future, poverty, fire, incurable illness.

■ **Extremely chilly; very sensitive to drafts and cold air**, may wrap up even in summer. Catches cold easily, especially in winter: ear discharges, cold sores and lymphatic enlargements are common.

■ **Skin unhealthy; may crack, peel and bleed**, particularly around the fingers. Sweats profusely, especially hands and feet. **Many eruptions**: pimples, vesicles, crusts, boils. **Pronounced tendency to itch**, better from cool air, and aggravated by washing, contact with wool, at night and the warmth of the bed; may scratch until it bleeds.

■ **Poor assimilation of food.** Loss of weight despite good appetite. Voracious hunger, especially at night, but may feel full after a few mouthfuls. Avoids fat, sugar, meat and coffee; loathes pork. **Thirsty**, especially for beer and acid drinks.

■ **Worse   Cold.** Outdoors. Drafts. Changes in weather. Storms. Menses.

Better   Warmth, except the skin itch. Wrapping up. Eating. Lying down.

Pulsatilla

ANEMONE PULSATILLA; WIND FLOWER

APPEARANCE

Often female. Light hair, blue eyes and a freckled face, tending to congestion and puffiness. Obesity and edema of the ankles are common. Movement may be clumsy; may stumble when walking. Tongue may be coated thickly white. Skin may be mottled.

SYMPTOM PICTURE

■ **Mild, gentle, yielding disposition**, shy and easily hurt, crying readily. May weep when telling symptoms. **Seeks sympathy and consolation, averse to solitude.** All symptoms are **changeable**; moods alter often, pains shift from place to place, menses are intermittent.

■ **Catarrhal discharge, from any mucous membrane**, yellow or greenish yellow, sticky and usually bland. Nasal discharge may alternate sides, is freer outdoors, and becomes blocked at night and in a warm room. **Seeks open air, even though chilly.** There may be **loss of smell and taste.**

■ **Periods irregular or intermittent**, with cramping and bearing down. **Thick yellowish leucorrhea**, slightly irritant.

■ **Often has no thirst.** May crave pastries, fat, ice cream and rich foods, which all disagree, or may avoid them completely. **Cream** in particular may upset. Prefers cool food and drink.

■ **Worse Heat.** Warm rooms. Rest. Evenings.

Better Consolation. Cool, open air. Gentle movement. Cold applications.

Keywords

Changeable
Tearful
Better company and consolation

Ranunculus Bulbosus

BULBOUS BUTTERCUP

APPEARANCE

Red cheeks, and a preference for stillness, because any movement will increase suffering.

SYMPTOM PICTURE

■ Overexcitable and oversensitive in the mornings, easily irritable and quarrelsome. **Great sensitivity to touch, cold and drafts.** Depression, with desire to die. Bad effects of alcoholism.

■ Eruption of **vesicles** with **intense itching, stinging and burning**, worse by cold and touch, even pressure of the clothes. A remedy for **shingles.**

■ Acute **shooting pains in chest wall and between ribs**, worse by touch and movement. Pleurisy. Intercostal neuralgia.

■ **Hay fever**, with smarting and burning in the eyes. **Constant tingling and crawling sensation** in the nose or nasopharynx, with ineffectual hawking to gain relief.

■ **Worse** Movement. Touch. Wet, cold weather. Changes in weather.

Better Sitting down. Leaning forward.

Keywords

Sensitive
Itching
Stinging
Shooting

Rhododendron Ferrugineum

ALPINE ROSE

APPEARANCE

There may be unequal pupils and rheumatic nodules. The tongue may be coated and greenish.

SYMPTOM PICTURE

■ **Anxious, depressed and nervous**, with a sensitivity to storms and a fear of thunder. Apathetic; averse to effort of any kind. Memory impaired; loses the thread when talking, and omits words when writing. Vertigo.

■ **Pains tearing, aching and jerking; can be anywhere**, but always **worse before a storm and immediately relieved by movement.** Pains come and go, and shift from one place to another; may drive from bed at night. **Stiffness and swelling** often in forearms, fingers, legs and toes. Wrists feel as if sprained. Gout.

■ **Coldness of the extremities**, even in a warm room; hands may feel hot but are cold to touch. Sweats, profuse and debilitating, with itching and tingling.

■ Testicles retracted, swollen and painful, even without infection.

■ **Worse Before storms.** Cold, wet and windy weather. Night. Rest.

Better Motion. Warmth. After storms.

Keywords

Stiff
Sore and swollen
Worse before storms

Rhus Toxicodendron

RHUS TOX; POISON IVY

APPEARANCE

Face may be suffused, with a red flush and a flaming red nose, or pale and sickly, with sunken eyes surrounded by blue rings. Restless; cannot sit or lie still for long. The tongue may have a triangular red tip.

SYMPTOM PICTURE

■ **Restlessness of mind**, with depression, sadness and apprehension about the future. Desire for solitude. May weep without knowing why. **Chilly**, with great sensitivity to open air or uncovering.

■ **Painful stiffness in bone, muscle or connective tissue**, often after overstrain or getting wet while hot. **Great restlessness** of body, even when exhausted. **Pains worse in bed at night, and on beginning to move, but better on continued motion.**

■ **Eruptions**, may be vesicular or crusty, **burning and itching**, especially around the scalp, face and genitals. Edema is common. Sweats may be persistent and offensive.

■ **Great thirst for cold drinks**, especially milk at night, with dryness of mouth, throat and tongue. Dislike of milk and bread.

■ **Worse   Damp cold. At the beginning of movement. Humidity. Rest.**

  Better   Heat. Continued, slow movement. Changes in position.

Keywords

Restless
Stiff and painful
Worse still
Better moving

Ruta Graveolens

RUTA GRAV; RUE

APPEARANCE

The eyes may look tired, red and watery. There may be a red rash on the forehead or pimples on the lips. Yawning is frequent. Restlessness may be obvious. The gait may be unsteady and staggering.

SYMPTOM PICTURE

■ **Restlessness** of mind, with anxiety, as if from a troubled conscience. Peevish, may be quarrelsome. Depressed at sundown. **Chilly**, and prefers indoors.

■ **Stiffness and pain in the limbs and joints**, as if after a fall, with **bruised weakness and weariness.** Tenderness and pain in muscles, or at the insertion of ligament and tendon into membrane covering bone. **Restlessness and uneasiness of the limbs**, especially the legs; does not know where to put them for relief. Lameness after sprains.

■ **Eyestrain** and eye fatigue, particularly after fine work, with redness, blurred vision, heat and burning.

■ Poor appetite, with easy satiety. Insatiable thirst for cold water. Meat and milk disagree.

■ **Worse   Cold and wet.** Rest. Lying on the painful part. Walking outdoors.

Better   Movement. Warmth.

Keywords

Weak
Bruised
Stiff
Strained

Sabadilla

SCHOENOCAULON OFFICINALE

APPEARANCE
Chilly and well wrapped up.

SYMPTOM PICTURE

■ Tendency to illusions and imaginary problems: Imagines that limbs are twisted, or that skin is wrinkled. **Hypersensitive** to the smell of garlic and flowers. **Chilly**; very sensitive to cold rooms, cold drinks and cold foods.

■ **Tonsillitis on left side**, or beginning on the left and spreading to the right, helped by hot drinks. **Itching of the throat**; tries to touch the throat with his or her tongue.

■ **Hay fever, especially from flowers**, with tickling in the throat. Fits of sneezing, with copious watery nasal discharge. Sensation of burning, itching or blockage in the nose, helped by hot air. Streaming eyes, red and burning.

■ Loathing for food and no thirst, but craves sweets. Itching of the anus, alternating with itching of the nose and ears. A remedy for pinworms, roundworms and tapeworms.

■ **Worse   Cold.** Full moon.

   Better   Heat. Hot drinks. Hot food.

Keywords

Chilly
Sneezing
Throat sore
Itching

Sabina

JUNIPERUS SABINA; SAVINE

APPEARANCE
Often female.

SYMPTOM PICTURE

■ Irritable and hypochondriacal. Cannot stand music: sets the nerves on edge. Hot flushes, with desire for open windows.

■ **Periods** early, heavy and prolonged, with **violent and piercing pains** moving from sacrum to pubis and the upper thighs, or cutting upwards into the vagina. Discharge of **bright red blood, mixed with clots, gushes on the least movement.** A remedy for threatened miscarriage at the third month.

■ **Warts and overgrowths**, can be anywhere, but especially **in the anal and genital area.** Warts itch and burn, and bleed easily.

■ Appetite is poor. There is a desire for juicy things, especially lemonade, and for sour things.

■ **Worse Heat. Movement.** Night. Bending forward.

Better Cold open air. Lying on back.

Keywords

Warts
Bleeds
Pains violent and
piercing

Sanguinaria Canadensis

BLOOD ROOT

Often young people, or women at menopause. Red cheeks and red ears; dilated veins in the temples. Palms and soles appear dry and wrinkled. The breath may be offensive.

SYMPTOM PICTURE

■ **Languor and torpor**, with no motivation for effort of any kind. The mood varies: is often anxious, but can be morose, irritable, peevish or excited.

■ **Congestive headache and periodic migraine**, with throbbing pains, usually on the right side. **Hot flushes over the face**, with redness of the ears, especially at menopause. **Intense burning of the palms and soles**; puts feet out of bed.

■ Prone to catching cold. **Hay fever, with burning** dryness of the nose and throat, changing to **sneezing with profuse burning secretion**. There may be increased sensitivity to smells, or complete loss of smell and taste.

■ Digestive disturbance with burning often accompanies other symptoms; **often must belch or pass wind for relief**. Sinking, "all-gone" sensation in stomach, without desire for food, especially in the morning. **Unquenchable thirst, with desire for acid and spicy things**. Averse to butter and sweets.

■ **Worse**   Cold and damp. Touch or jar. Periodically, every day, second day or week. Right side.

Better   Lying on left side. Sleep. Belching. Passing wind.

Keywords

Burning
Thirsty
Flushing
Acrid

Sepia

INK FROM THE CUTTLEFISH

SYMPTOM PICTURE

■ **Tired, worn-out, pessimistic and indifferent.** Easily moved to tears; may weep when telling symptoms. Hysterical, irritable and quarrelsome, with fear of not coping and losing control. **Indifferent to family:** can reject those most loved. **Averse to consolation. Seeks solitude, yet fears it.**

■ **Premenstrual tension.** Menstruation with **sensation of heaviness and dragging down,** especially in the uterus; may want to sit down and cross legs. Leucorrhea yellow–green, offensive and irritant, making the vagina dry and painful during intercourse. Often averse to sex.

■ **Usually chilly,** but sweats easily in armpits, back and genitals. **Hot flushes, especially at menopause,** without much redness, but with sweating and fainting. Better from vigorous exercise, especially dancing.

■ Appetite varies; may have ravenous hunger or anorexia. Sinking feeling about 11 a.m. May crave vinegar, pickles and acid foods. May be averse to meat, milk and fat. **In pregnancy, nausea at the sight or smell of food.**

■ **Worse** Consolation. Cold. Standing still. Menstruation, pregnancy and lactation. Forenoon and evening.

Better **Vigorous exercise.** Open air and wind. Warmth of bed.

Keywords

Weary
Heavy
Indifferent
Sad
Chilly
Irritable

Spongia Tosta

ROASTED SEA SPONGE

APPEARANCE

Fair, with light-colored hair and blue eyes. Timid and sensitive children. There may be a flushed face and restricted breathing.

SYMPTOM PICTURE

■ **Marked anxiety**, even terror in most complaints, and generally associated with **suffocative attacks**. Extreme exhaustion and heaviness of the body after even slight exhaustion. **Chilly**, especially in the back.

■ **Raucous, dry, barking cough**, like a saw through wood, with suffocative attacks. **Anxious wheezing**, with constriction and burning, **worse during inspiration. Croup.** Whooping cough. Asthma.

■ **Cardiac disturbance**, with palpitations, suffocation and anxiety. Angina, worse from motion, ascending and at night.

■ **Enlargement and induration of the thyroid**, with palpitations, suffocative attacks on exertion and at night. Enlargement of lymph nodes and salivary glands.

■ **Worse** **Around midnight.** Lying with the head down. Cold drinks.

   Better **Hot drinks.** Lying with the head up. Sitting up and bending forward.

Keywords

Anxious
Suffocative
Dry
Barking
Croupy

Staphysagria

DELPHINIUM STAPHISAGRIA; STAVESACRE

APPEARANCE

May have a sickly look, with sunken, blue-ringed eyes. Children have a scrawny, pot-bellied appearance.

SYMPTOM PICTURE

■ Cultivated and polite, **controlling feelings at any price**, but **easily offended** and **silently brooding** over wrongs, either real or imaginary. **Suppressed anger and indignation**, resulting in **resentment**, indifference, poor memory and insomnia. Child is cross and demanding but refuses things when offered, pushes them away.

■ **Great sensitivity** to noise, tastes and odors, **but particularly to pain**, with **burning and prickling pains** in any organ, aggravated by touch. A remedy for surgical wounds or cuts, and for decaying teeth.

■ **Frequent urination, with burning pains when not urinating. Dwells on sexual matters**; may be impotent. Exhausted by sexual excess and masturbation. **Genital warts.**

■ **Eczema** of face, scalp and eyelids, with thick crusts and irritating, weeping lesions, forming new vesicles on contact. **Styes and cysts of the eyelids.** Pedunculated warts, may be either dry or moist.

■ **Worse** Anger, indignation and disappointment. Sexual excess. Cold. Least touch.
Better Warmth. Rest. After a meal.

Keywords

Sensitive
Suppressed
Resentful
Burning
Prickling

Sulphur

APPEARANCE

May be lean and hungry looking, or fat and rotund. Red face, red ears, freckles and a red tip on the nose are common. The skin is dry, rough and scaly. Hair tends to be coarse and lusterless. Hands are hot and sweaty.

SYMPTOM PICTURE

■ Hale, hearty and self-confident when well; becomes selfish, stubborn, irritable and critical when ill. **Absent-minded**; poor memory for names and recent events, but **enjoys philosophy, anecdote or argument.** Intelligent with periods of brilliance, but lack of staying power. Tendency to bluff.

■ **Heat and burning** in any part of the body, but especially **in the crown of the skull, palms and soles**, with redness of body orifices and **intolerance of heat. Hot flushes,** especially at menopause.

■ Rough, dry, scaly skin, **itches and burns, worse from heat and bathing.** Uncontrollable desire to scratch, which improves for a while, then worsens. Secretions are burning, irritating and offensive. Usually a lack of sweat.

■ Notable hunger except in morning. Thirst for large amounts of water. Sinking feeling around 11 a.m. Craving for **sweets**, spices, fats, salt, pickles and alcohol, but can be averse to them. Averse to eggs and milk.

■ **Worse Heat. Standing. Water. Night. 11 a.m. Drafts. After sleep.**

Better Warm, dry weather. Free elimination. **Movement.** Cool, fresh air.

Keywords

Hot
Burning
Forgetful
Worse heat

Tabacum

TOBACCO LEAF

APPEARANCE

Face pale, blue and pinched. There may be a cold sweat.

SYMPTOM PICTURE

■ **Deathly nausea and vomiting**, with pale face, **salivation, cold sweat** and complete prostration, worse by motion and heat, and better by fresh air and closing the eyes. A remedy for **travel sickness** and **morning sickness.**

■ **Vertigo, with death-like pallor**, increasing to loss of consciousness, relieved in open air or by vomiting. Headache, beginning in the morning and intolerable by noon, with nausea and violent vomiting.

■ **Cardiac disturbances.** Violent palpitations. Angina, with pale face, cold sweat, nausea and vomiting.

■ Diarrhea, sudden and urgent, with nausea, vomiting and prostration. Constipation, with inactive bowel and spasms of the sphincter.

■ **Worse   Motion.** Heat.

Better   Fresh air. Rest. Closing eyes.

Keywords

Pale
Cold
Sweating
Salivating
Nauseous
Prostrated

Thuja Occidentalis

WHITE CEDAR

APPEARANCE

Excessive hairiness and obesity, with heavy trunk, short neck, thin limbs, waxy, greasy skin and irregular teeth, but the skin and hair may also be fine and the features delicate.

There may be a red capillary network on the sides of the nose, and ridges or streaks on the nails.

SYMPTOM PICTURE

■ **Easy exhaustion, with anxiety.** Truthful and scrupulous; often very polite in public, but **obsessive, depressed, impatient and irritable** in private. Affectionate, but averse to touch; dislike of strangers. **Fixed ideas.**

■ **Disorders of mucous membranes**, especially urinary tract, genitals and lung. Chronic catarrh, irritating and profuse, a **yellow–green discharge**, with odor often suggestive of **fish-brine, garlic or honey.** Asthma, around 3 a.m.

■ **Moles, warts, polyps, scaly eruptions** and other overgrowths of the skin. **Chilly,** and sensitive to damp, with tearing pains in the muscles and joints, and deposits in the joints. Profuse sweat on uncovered parts, with foul or sweetish smell.

■ Appetite is poor, with easy satiety after a few mouthfuls; often no desire for breakfast. Prefers cold food and craves salt. Averse to onions. Thirst is not marked, but may have to drink with meals to facilitate swallowing.

■ **Worse** Damp and humidity. Cold. 3 a.m. and 3 p.m. Heat of the bed. Morning.

Better Heat. Sweating.

Keywords

Chilly
Anxious
Irritable
Stiff
Warty
Worse from damp

Urtica

URTICA URENS; NETTLE

APPEARANCE
Not defined.

SYMPTOM PICTURE

■ A remedy with its best use in **burning, stinging, blotchy rashes**, often with severe itching. Hence it covers **hives, nettle rash, prickly heat** and some **insect bites.** It is often the remedy to antidote an **allergic reaction to eating shellfish.**

■ **Minor burns**, with burning, stinging pains afterwards.

■ Rheumatic **pains in the joints, swollen, burning and stinging**, with constant desire to rub the skin. Gout.

■ A useful remedy for **breastfeeding** mothers, when the **milk supply is low or overabundant.** It will act as a normaliser, and will also assist in arresting the flow of milk after weaning.

■ **Worse** Cold applications. Bathing. Washing.

Better Rubbing.

Keywords

Rashes

Bites

Burns

Burning

Itching and stinging

Veratrum Album

WHITE HELLEBORE

APPEARANCE

In the acute case the face is pale or bluish, eyes sunken, features drawn, and has an expression of anguish or fear. The facial muscles may jerk or twitch. The body is cold to touch, with cold sweat apparent on the face.

SYMPTOM PICTURE

■ Restless activity, must be constantly occupied. Fits of mania, with hysteria, loquacity and muttering; may become obscene. Inconsolable, yet fears solitude. May come as the result of fright, emotional trauma, shock or injury, even from resentment. Delirium and hallucinations. Neuralgic pains, can be anywhere, driving frantic.

■ **Collapse with coldness and blueness**, with cold sweat, especially on the forehead, and deathly pallor. In less severe cases, fainting may occur from emotional stress or exertion.

■ **Profuse discharges** with rapid exhaustion and prostration. **Acute, violent vomiting or purging.** Copious sweat, urine and saliva. Period pain, with vomiting and purging.

■ **Intense thirst**, with desire for large quantities of cold drinks, or ice to suck. Violent hunger, with craving for cold food and aversion to hot food. Intolerance of fruit.

■ **Worse** Heat. Damp cold weather. Movement. Pressure.

Better Rest. Coolness.

Keywords

Cold
Blue
Sweating
Vomiting
Purging

Zincum Metallicum

ZINC

APPEARANCE

Pale, weak and tired, slow to understand and speak because of exhaustion. There may be fine twitching of the muscles. The feet may move continually when sitting, or the head when lying down.

SYMPTOM PICTURE

■ **Slowness and exhaustion** arising from illness, overwork and overstress, drunkenness, insomnia or fright. **Oversensitive**, nervous and excitable; can jump at the least noise, and **easily irritated** by trifles. **Unable to relax**, with trembling, jerking and twitching of muscles.

■ **Ailments from inability to initiate a discharge**, but **improved when it appears.** Discharges can be anywhere: teething, menses, skin eruptions, urine, expectoration. **Ailments from suppressed discharges.**

■ **Chilly**, especially when outdoors, **yet sweats easily** on the slightest exertion. **Night sweats**, can be profuse and continuous.

■ **Weak, "all-gone" feeling about 11 a.m.**, often provokes ravenous hunger. Averse to sugar, milk, meat and fish. The least amount of wine may cause headache or flushing. Thirst may be extreme, especially in the afternoon.

■ **Worse** Exertion. Noise. Wine and stimulants. 11 a.m. to noon. Before discharge, eruption or elimination.

Better Appearance of discharge.

Keywords

Restless
Tired and twitching
Worse before
discharges

13

A Home Medicine Kit

*H*ere is a list of commonly used remedies. You will be able to obtain most of them from health food shops, but major suppliers are listed.

REMEDY	COMMON SYMPTOMS
Aconite	Fever and inflammation. Cough. Earache. Croup.
Apis	Sore throats. Insect bites and stings. Itching, burning skin.
Arnica	Bruises, bumps and thumps. Muscular aches and overstrains.
Arsenicum	Inflammation and pain with burning, worse around midnight.
Belladonna	Fever. Earache. Sore throat. Scarlet fever. Mumps.
Bryonia	Sore throat. Fever. Coughs and colds. Influenza.
Calc fluor	A tissue salt for bones, teeth and skin, varicose veins and piles.
Calc phos	A tissue salt for growth, bones and teeth, and cramps.

Calc sulp	A tissue salt for skin suppuration, wounds, yellow discharges.
Calendula	Cuts and septic wounds, with bright blood.
Camphor	Sensation of icy cold. Collapse.
Capsicum	Inflammation of the throat, nose and ear.
Carbo veg	Digestive bloating and flatulence. Collapse. Craving for fresh air.
Chamomilla	Irritability, teething, colic, insomnia. Digestive upsets.
China	Exhaustion, digestive disorders.
Cocculus	Exhaustion, nausea, travel sickness. Collapse.
Coffea	Insomnia, with great mental activity.
Eupatorium	Influenza with bone pain.
Ferrum phos	A tissue salt for fever and inflammation.
Gelsemium	Influenza and sore throats, developing slowly. Jet lag.
Hamamelis	Bruising, with dark blood.
Hepar sulph	Sore throat. Coughs and colds. Croup. Septic wounds.
Hypericum	Jammed fingers. Sprains. Puncture wounds.
Ignatia	Emotional upsets. Spasms, cramps and twitches. Insomnia.
Kali mur	A tissue salt for coughs and colds with white discharges.
Kali phos	A tissue salt for exhaustion, stress, irritability and insomnia.
Kali sulph	A tissue salt for yellow discharges, coughs and skin problems.
Ledum	Puncture wounds. Insect bites and stings.
Mag phos	A tissue salt for muscular cramps, spasms and pain.
Mercurius	Influenza, sore throat. Mumps.
Nat mur	A tissue salt for colds, cold sores and fluid imbalance.
Nat phos	A tissue salt for acid conditions and creamy discharges.
Nat sulph	A tissue salt for bilious conditions and fluid retention.

Nux vomica	Irritability, stress and insomnia. Constipation. Hangovers.
Pulsatilla	Earache. Measles. Cough. PMS. Emotional upsets.
Rhus tox	Influenza. Chickenpox. Muscular pain better by motion.
Ruta grav	Strains and sprains. Repetitive strain injury.
Sepia	PMS. Menstrual discomfort. Emotional upsets. Exhaustion.
Silicea	A tissue salt for fatigue, and for poor skin, hair and nails.
Spongia	Cough. Croup.
Staphysagria	Excessive irritability. Styes. Stinging wounds.
Veratrum album	Collapse. Vomiting, diarrhea, prostration.

TINCTURES	COMMON SYMPTOMS
Arnica	Bruises and sprains when the skin is unbroken.
Calendula	Lacerated tissue, septic wounds.
Hamamelis	Bruises and sprains when the skin is broken.
Hypericum	Cuts and septic wounds. Jammed fingers.
Ledum	Puncture wounds, insect bites.
Urtica	Burns. Stings. Rashes. Hives.

Resource Guide of Suppliers

*M*ost health food stores and chains, and many pharmacies, carry more or less comprehensive selections of homeopathic remedies. Some firms offer homeopathic products from a variety of manufacturers by mail order (as well, often, as in a store). Here is a brief list of some such firms.

L&H Vitamins, Inc.,
32–33 47th Avenue
Long Island City, NY 11101
1-800-221-1152

National Homeopathic Products
518 Tasman Street, Suite B
Madison, WI 53714
1-800-888-4066
 (also a manufacturer)

Penn Herb Co.
603 North 2nd Street
Philadelphia, PA 19123
215 925-3336
 (also a manufacturer)

Santa Monica Homeopathic Pharmacy
629 Broadway
Santa Monica, CA 90401
310 395-1131

Vitamin Power
39 St. Mary's Place
Freeport, NY 11520
1-800-645-6587

Vitamin Shoppe
4700 Westside Avenue
North Bergen, NJ 07407
1-800-223-1216

Willner Chemists
330 Lexington Avenue
New York, NY 10016
212 685-0448
1-800-633-1106

MANUFACTURERS

There are more than 50 manufacturers of homeopathic remedies in the
United States; here is a brief listing of some of the better-known ones. Most
manufacturers will provide information about their products and where they
can be purchased, but do not handle retail sales, though some will.

Boericke & Tafel
2381 Circadian Way
Santa Rosa, CA 95407-5439
707 571-8202
1-800-876-9505

Boiron
6 Campus Boulevard, Building A
Newton Square, PA 19073-3200
610 325-746

Ellon USA, Inc.
644 Merrick Road
Lynbrook, NY 11563-2332
516 593-2206
1-800-423-2556

Dolisos America Homeopathy
3014 Rigel Avenue
Las Vegas, NV 89102-0718
702 871-7153
1-800-365-4767

Enzymatic Therapy
825 Challenger Drive
Green Bay, WI 54311-8328
414 469-1313

Nature's Way
PO Box 4000
Springville, UT 84663-9007
801 489-1500

Nelson Bach USA Ltd
1007 West Upsal Street
Philadelphia, PA 19119-3716
215 844-2224
1-800-314-BACH

Sunsource Health Products, Inc.
535 Lipoa Parkway, Suite 110
Kihei, HI 96753-6902
808 879-6864
1-800-446-7262

Bibliography and Acknowledgments

I am happy to acknowledge my indebtedness to the following authors for their works, which have been used as general references in the compilation of this book.

HOMEOPATHIC REMEDIES

Boericke, William, *Materia Medica with Repertory*, B. Jain Publishers, New Delhi, 1988

Boger, C.M., *Synoptic Key of the Materia Medica*, B. Jain Publishers, New Delhi, 1931

Borland, Douglas, *Homoeopathy in Practice*, Beaconsfield Publishers, Beaconsfield, Hampshire UK, 1982

Boyd, Hamish, *Introduction to Homoeopathic Medicine*, Beaconsfield Publishers, Beaconsfield, Hampshire, UK, 1979

Darragh, Frances and Louise, *Healing Your Child*, New Women's Press, Auckland, 1989

Gemmell, David, *Everyday Homoeopathy*, Beaconsfield Publishers, Beaconsfield, Hampshire, UK, 1987

Gibson, Douglas, *Studies of Homoeopathic Remedies*, Beaconsfield Publishers, Beaconsfield, Hampshire, UK, 1987

Golden, Isaac, *Australian Homoeopathic Home Prescriber*, Martin and Pleasance, Richmond, Victoria, 1993

Jouanny, Jacques, *The Essentials of the Homoeopathic Materia Medica*, Laboratoires Boiron, Bordeaux, 1980

King, Ken, *Lectures on Homoeopathic Miasms*, unpublished material

Lockie, *The Family Guide to Homoeopathy*, Book Club Associates, 1991

Mathur, Kailash, *Systematic Materia Medica of Homoeopathic Remedies*, B. Jain Publishers, New Delhi, 1979

Tyler, M.L., *Pointers to the Common Remedies*, B. Jain Publishers, New Delhi, 1980

TISSUE SALTS

Martin and Pleasance, *Handbook of the Biochemic Tissue Salts*, Desktop Publishing, Richmond, Victoria 1991

Schuessler, William, *Biochemic Handbook*, New Era Laboratories, London, 1975

BACH FLOWER REMEDIES

Bach, Edward, *Heal Thyself*, C.W. Daniel, Saffron Waldon, Essex, 1931

————*The Twelve Healers*, C.W. Daniel, Saffron Waldon, Essex, 1933

Chancellor, Phillip, *Illustrated Handbook of the Bach Flower Remedies*, C.W. Daniel, Saffron Waldon, Essex, 1971

Wells, Mark, *The Bach Flower Remedies Today*, Autonomy Australia, Melbourne, 1993

$\mathcal{I}$ndex

NOTE: For illnesses, primary listing is differentiated from secondary mentions by **boldface**

Veratrum album 37, 39, 69, 76, 168, 324, 329

vertigo **129–30,** 229, 248, 273, 376, 304, 311, 321

Vibernum 73, 174, 175, 191

Vinca 137

Viola 137, 142

Vipera 129

voice, loss of **96–97,** 247, 251, 267

vomiting 40, 66, 71, 76, 77, 89, 90, 91, 98, 100, 105, 127, 128, **130–31,** 140, **144–45,** 148, 152, 153, 160, 163, 170–71, 225, 233, 244, 245, 273, 275, 276, 280, 292, 293, 321, 324, 329

warts **132,** 232, 234, 243, 244, 256, 267, 281, 302, 315, 319, 322

whooping cough 71, **162–63,** 271, 280, 318

worms, intestinal 271, 314

Zincum met 81, 173, 325

Paul Callinan began his career in science, taking his BSc in Physics, and then an MSc in Physiology at the University of Melbourne. He subsequently became interested in alternative medicine and trained as a homeopath, naturopath and chiropractor.

He now works as a lecturer, writer and research consultant to the natural therapies professions. He has been a contributing editor to *Wellbeing* magazine since its inception. He also runs his own natural therapies practice in Balgowlah, New South Wales, Australia.